@RosenTeenTalk

COPING WITH SOCIAL ANXIETY

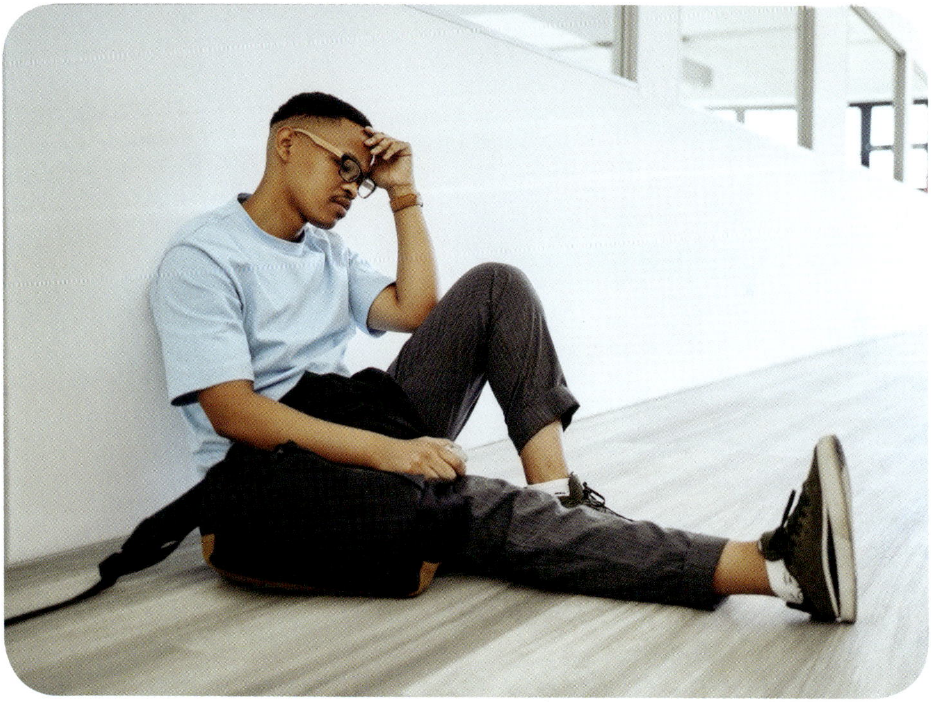

Katie Kawa

ROSEN PUBLISHING

Published in 2026 by The Rosen Publishing Group, Inc.
2544 Clinton Street, Buffalo, NY 14224

First Edition

Editor: Katie Kawa
Designer: Rachel Rising

Photo Credits: Cover, pp. 3, 4, 23, 45 PeopleImages.com - Yuri A/Shutterstock.com; Cover, Cosmic_Design/Shutterstock.com; Cover, pp. 1, 3-48 Vitya_M/Shutterstock.com; pp. 3,15, 25 fizkes/Shutterstock.com; pp. 3, 34 Ljupco Smokovski/Shutterstock.com; p. 6 kozhedub_nc/Shutterstock.com; p. 7 DimaBerlin/Shutterstock.com; p. 8 New Africa/Shutterstock.com; p. 9 SpeedKingz/Shutterstock.com; p. 10 Elena Kalinicheva/Shutterstock.com; p. 11 SynthEx/Shutterstock.com; p. 12 Amanda Alamsyah/Shutterstock.com; p. 13 Monkey Business Images/Shutterstock.com; p. 16 ProStockStudio/Shutterstock.com; p. 17 AYO Production/Shutterstock.com; p. 19 Raushan_films/Shutterstock.com; p. 20 GoodStudio/Shutterstock.com; p. 21 Andrey_Popov/Shutterstock.com; p. 22 KieferPix/Shutterstock.com; pp. 24, 27 Pixel-Shot/Shutterstock.com; p. 26 Alena Anisimova/Shutterstock.com; p. 28 Double Brain/Shutterstock.com; p. 29 EHStockphoto/Shutterstock.com; p. 30 Fahroni/Shutterstock.com; p. 31 Prathankarnpap/Shutterstock.com; p. 33 Media_Photos/Shutterstock.com; p. 35 InspireNest/Shutterstock.com; p. 36 KAMPUS/Shutterstock.com; p. 37 Prostock-studio/Shutterstock.com; p. 38 Edge Creative/Shutterstock.com; p. 39 Shift Drive/Shutterstock.com; p. 40 New Africa/Shutterstock.com; p. 41 fizkes/Shutterstock.com; p. 42 Sergey Furtaev/Shutterstock.com; p. 43 CarlosBarquero/Shutterstock.com.

Some of the images in this book illustrate individuals who are models. The depictions do not imply actual situations or events.

Library of Congress Cataloging-in-Publication Data

Names: Kawa, Katie author
Title: Coping with social anxiety / Katie Kawa.
Description: Buffalo, New York : Rosen Publishing, (2026) | Series: Rosenteentalk | Includes index.
Identifiers: LCCN 2025036962 | ISBN 9781725342552 library binding | ISBN 9781725342545 paperback | ISBN 9781725342569 ebook
Subjects: LCSH: Social phobia in adolescence--Juvenile literature
Classification: LCC RJ506.S63 K38 2026 | DDC 618.92/85225--dc23/eng/20250917
LC record available at https://lccn.loc.gov/2025036962

Manufactured in the United States of America

CPSIA Compliance Information: Batch #CWRYA26. For Further Information contact Rosen Publishing at 1-800-237-9932.

CONTENTS

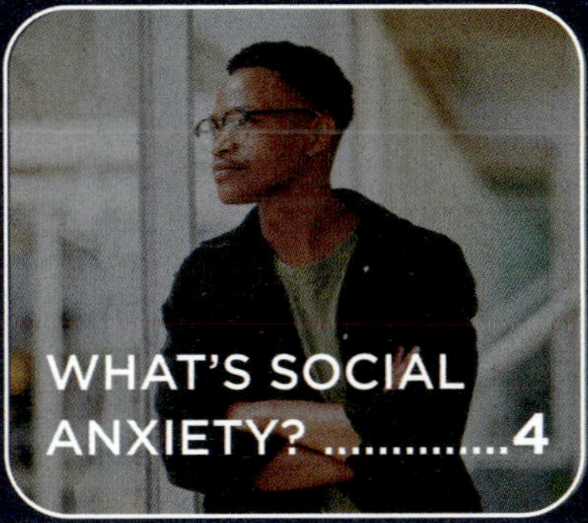
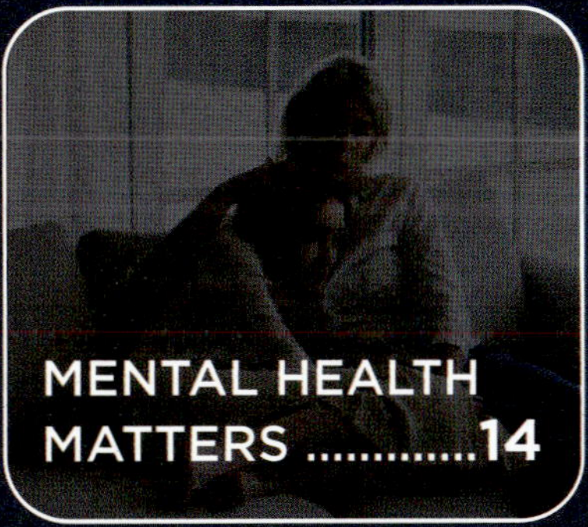
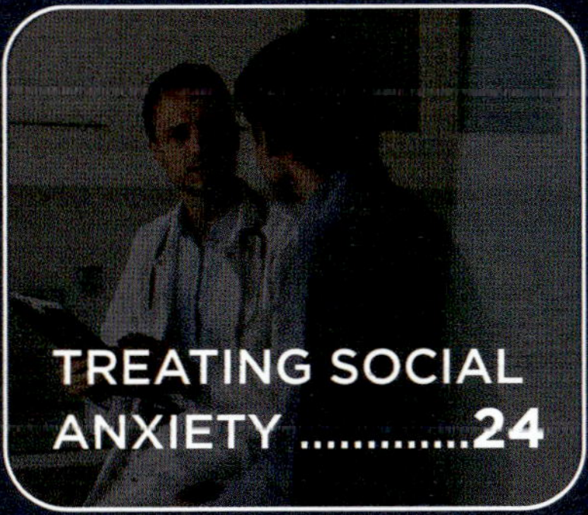
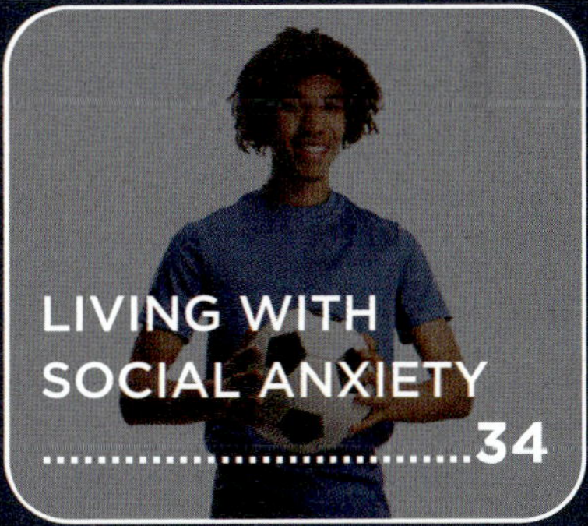

Chapter 1

What's Social Anxiety?

I've been having a really hard time at school lately. I hate being called on in class. What if I get the answer wrong and everyone laughs at me? What if I get it right and everyone calls me a know-it-all?

Lately, it's even been hard to be around my friends at lunch. I get so nervous eating in front of them. I worry that I'll get food on my face or I'll talk with my mouth full. I know my friends don't care about any of that, but I can't stop worrying.

It's gotten so bad that I feel sick on my way to school every day. My stomach hurts, and sometimes I start to feel really dizzy.

I don't want to feel like this! I think I need some help...

Social anxiety can make it hard for people to do everyday tasks, such as going to school or spending time with friends.

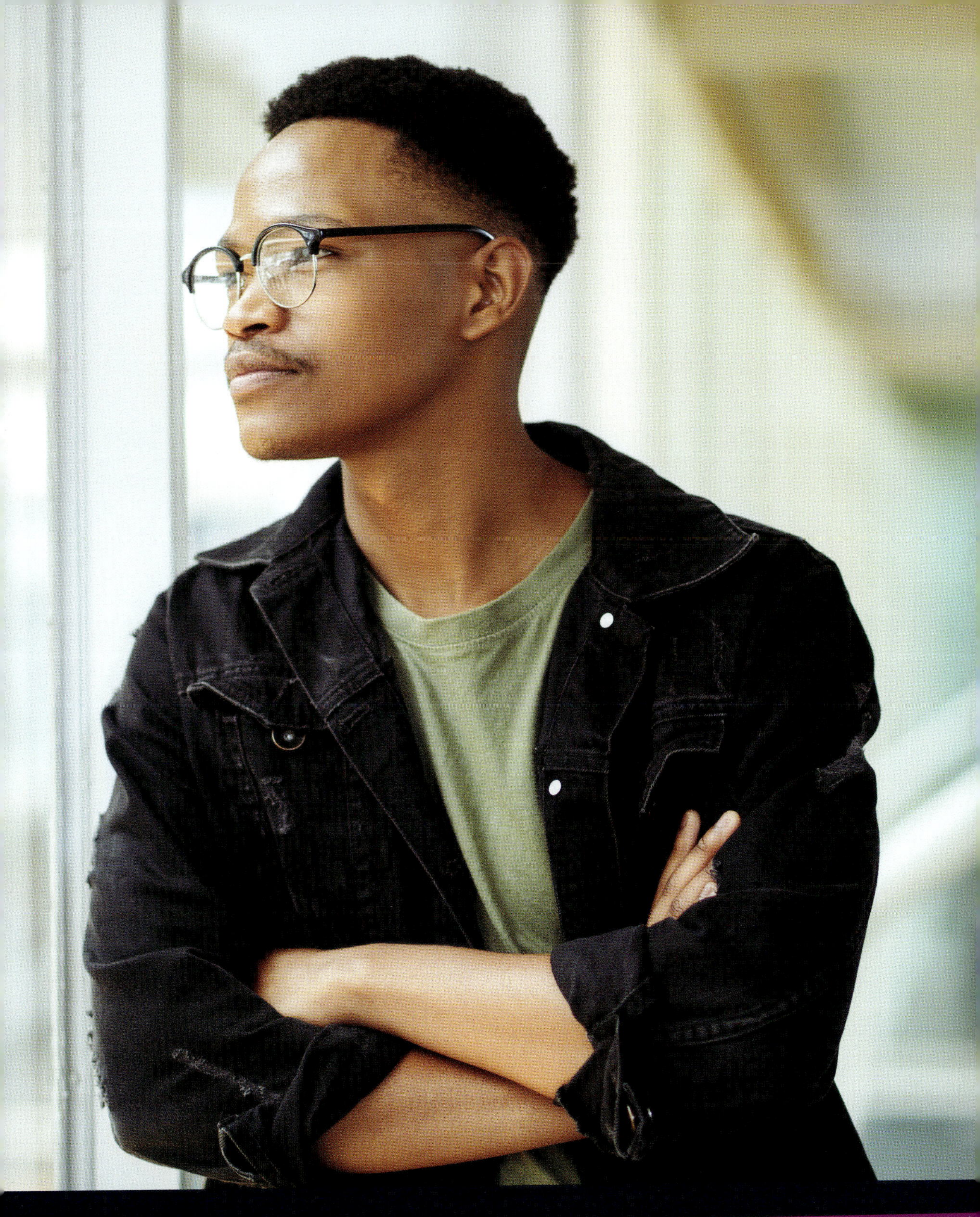

MORE THAN NORMAL NERVES

The first day at a new school, a job **interview**, a first date—these are all **situations** that can make a person feel anxious, or nervous and filled with worry. That's **normal**!

For some people, though, everyday situations, such as ordering at a restaurant or hanging out with a friend, cause the same kind of anxious feelings—or worse. These people live with social anxiety disorder. This is a **mental** health condition that causes people to feel overpowering anxiety about being watched or judged by others.

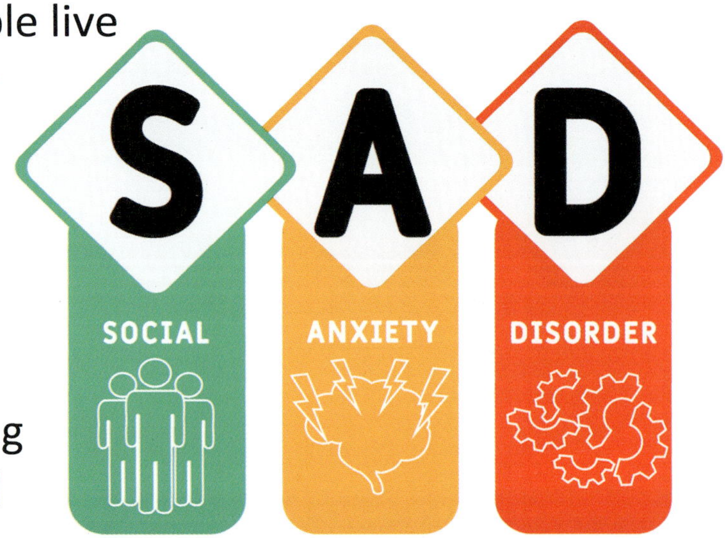

Fast Fact!

Around 7 percent of the U.S. population lives with social anxiety disorder. That's around 15 million people!

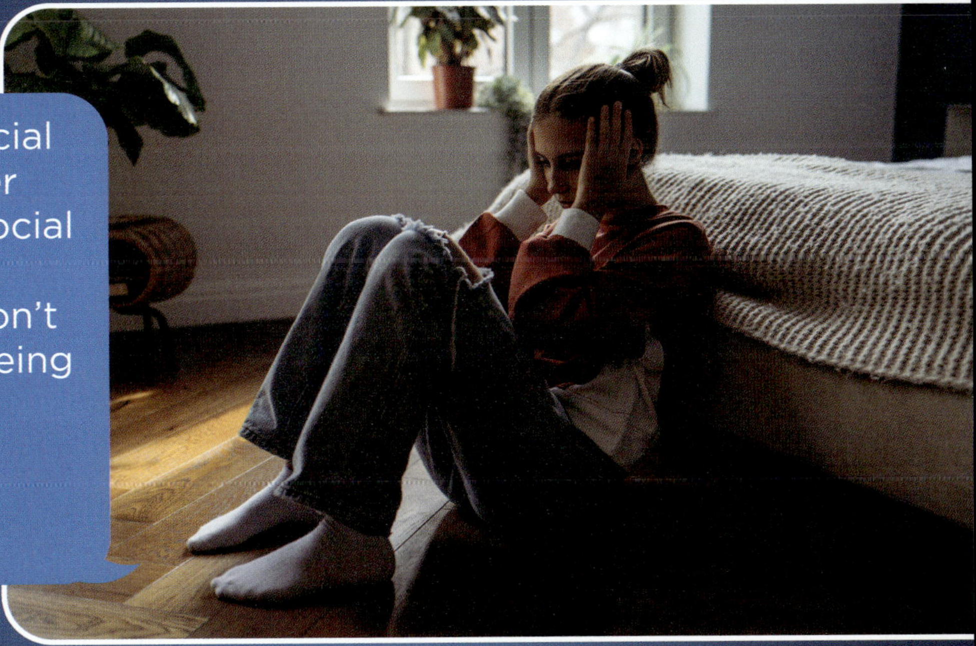

People with social anxiety disorder live in fear of social situations that most people don't worry about. Being around people causes them a lot of distress, or suffering.

WHAT IT'S NOT

Social anxiety disorder is not the same as shyness. When someone is shy, they might feel uncomfortable in social situations. However, their discomfort is not as **extreme** as the fear and worry felt by those with social anxiety disorder. In addition, having social anxiety isn't the same as being introverted. Introverts find big social events draining and recharge by being alone. However, they generally don't fear being around people the same way those with social anxiety disorder do.

COMMON WORRIES

At the core of social anxiety disorder is an extreme fear of being judged, laughed at, or **embarrassed**. This shows up in different ways for different people.

Many people with social anxiety disorder are afraid of looking **awkward** in front of others. They are often very self-conscious, or overly worried about how they appear to other people. In addition, they also tend to expect the worst when planning for a social situation. They often know these worries are **irrational**, but they can't stop them.

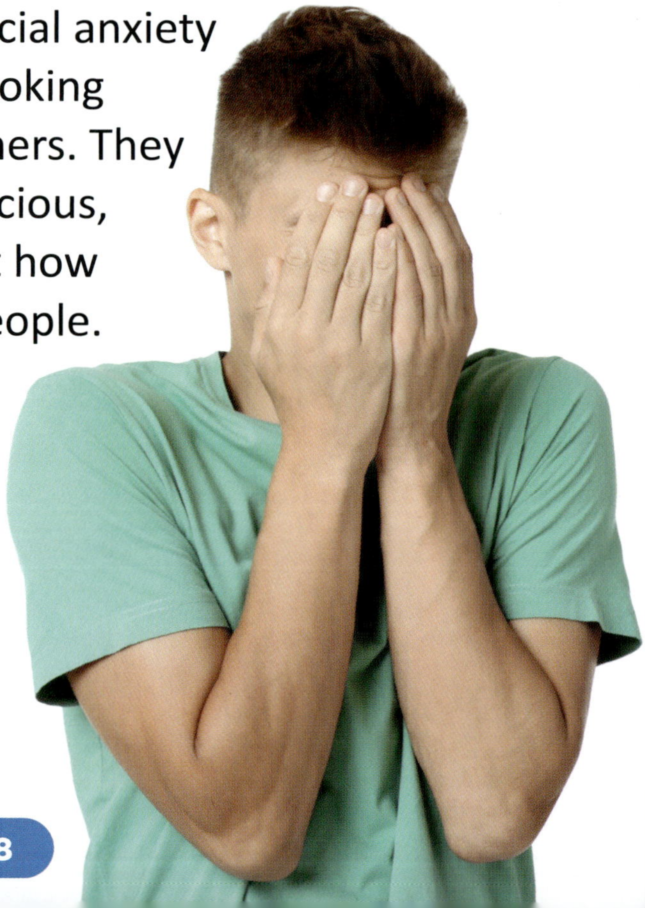

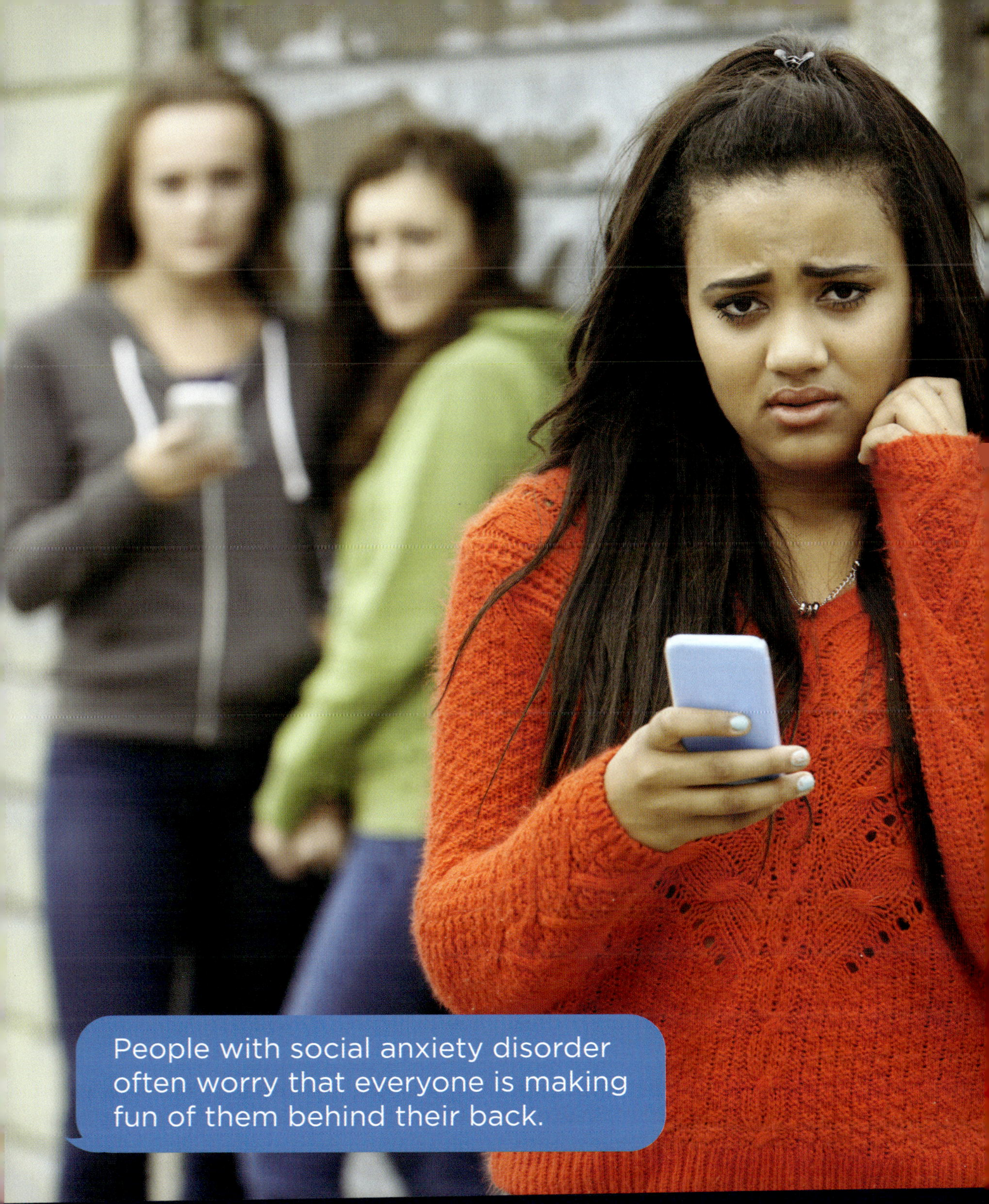

People with social anxiety disorder often worry that everyone is making fun of them behind their back.

PHYSICAL PROBLEMS

Social anxiety disorder often comes with many **physical** symptoms, or signs. These include things only the person dealing with them can feel—such as a fast heartbeat, dizziness, tight muscles, and stomach problems.

In addition, some symptoms of social anxiety disorder can be seen by others. These include blushing, sweating, and shaking. For many people with social anxiety disorder, these symptoms make their worries worse. They become afraid that everyone will know they're anxious, which they think is embarrassing.

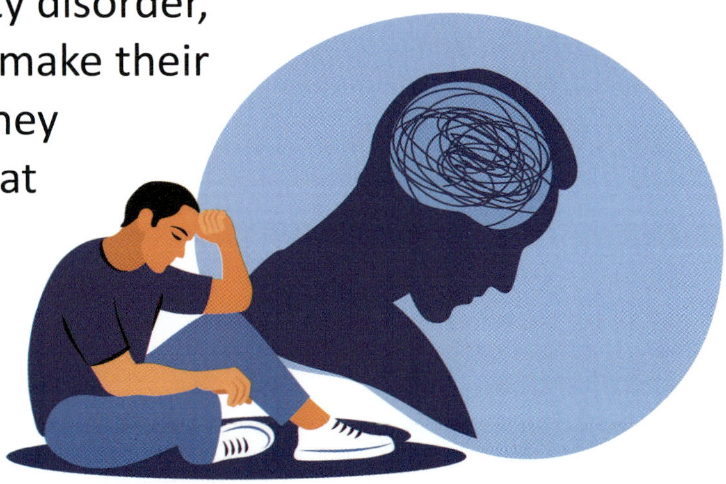

People with social anxiety disorder often have a hard time making direct eye contact with others, especially strangers.

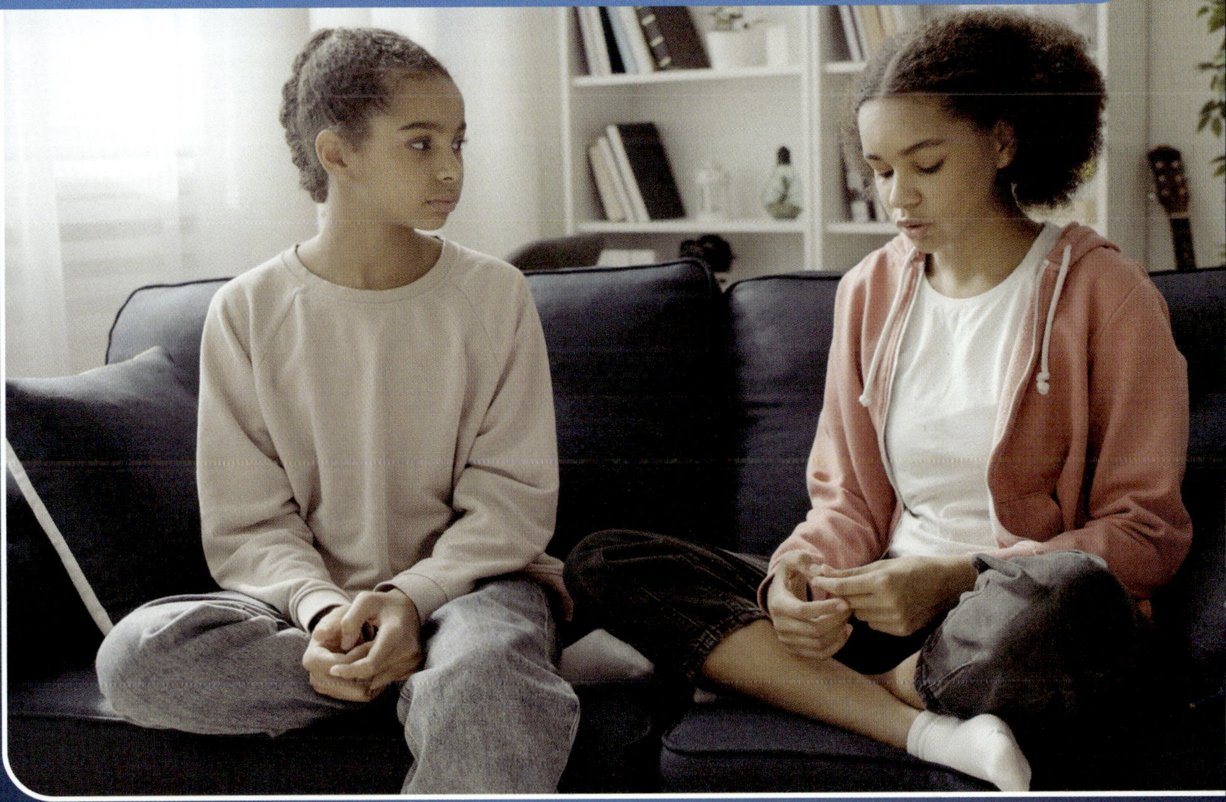

PANIC ATTACKS

In some cases, people with social anxiety disorder might have panic attacks. These are moments of extreme fear that happen very suddenly. This extreme fear causes physical symptoms, such as chest pain, sweating, **nausea**, and chills. A person's heart might beat very quickly, and they might have a hard time breathing. Someone having a panic attack might feel like they're dying but they aren't. Deep breathing and paying close attention to your surroundings can help if you're having a panic attack.

SCARY SITUATIONS

People with social anxiety disorder often feel so much distress and discomfort in social situations that they try to avoid them. They might avoid parties or other events where they might have to meet someone new. They might even cancel plans with friends or avoid answering the phone.

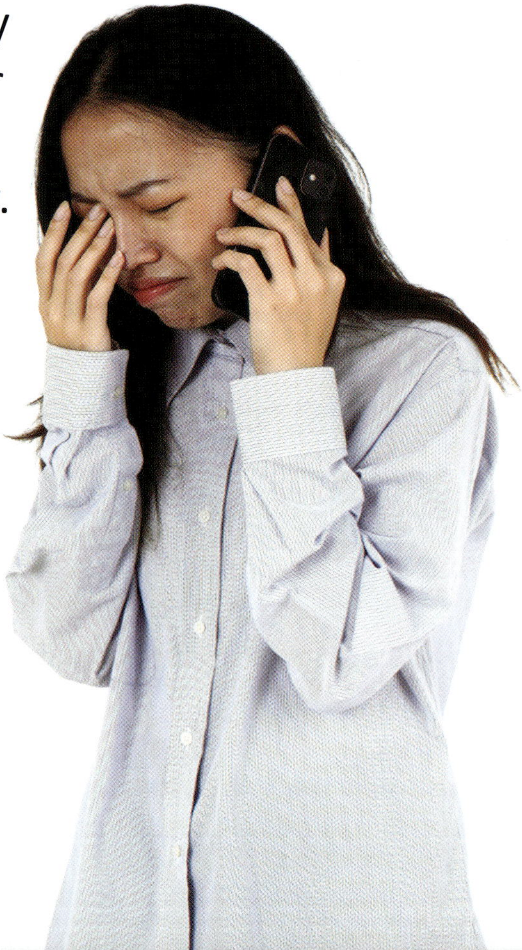

In some cases, social anxiety disorder can cause people to avoid going to school or work. It can even make it hard for people to go shopping or use a public bathroom.

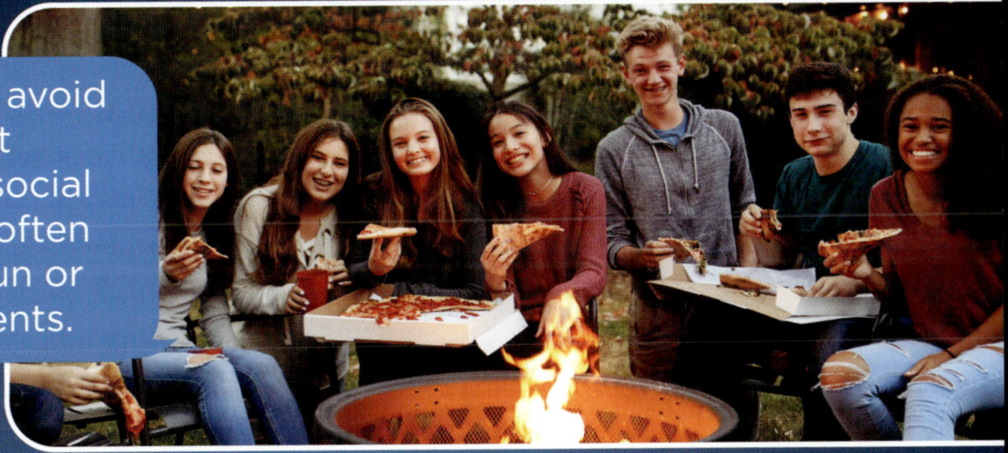

When people avoid situations that **trigger** their social anxiety, they often miss out on fun or important events.

WHAT ARE PEOPLE AFRAID OF?

Common social situations that can be scary for people with social anxiety disorder include:

- going to school or work
- meeting new people
- answering the phone or making a call
- eating in front of other people
- ordering at a restaurant
- asking for help at a store
- answering a question in class
- dating
- interviewing for a job
- using a public bathroom
- walking into a room full of people

Chapter 2

Mental Health Matters

My parents don't get it. I've been anxious around people for as long as I can remember, but it's gotten really bad the last couple of years. Whenever I have to talk to people, I start to sweat and my hands get really shaky.

I know it's normal to get nervous before giving a speech or asking someone on a date. But I start to panic when I order dinner at a restaurant or talk to my grandma on the phone. I get so worried I'm going to say something embarrassing that I want to hide just thinking about it.

My mom and dad tell me not to worry about what other people think of me. But it's not that easy!

Telling someone with an anxiety disorder not to worry isn't very helpful.

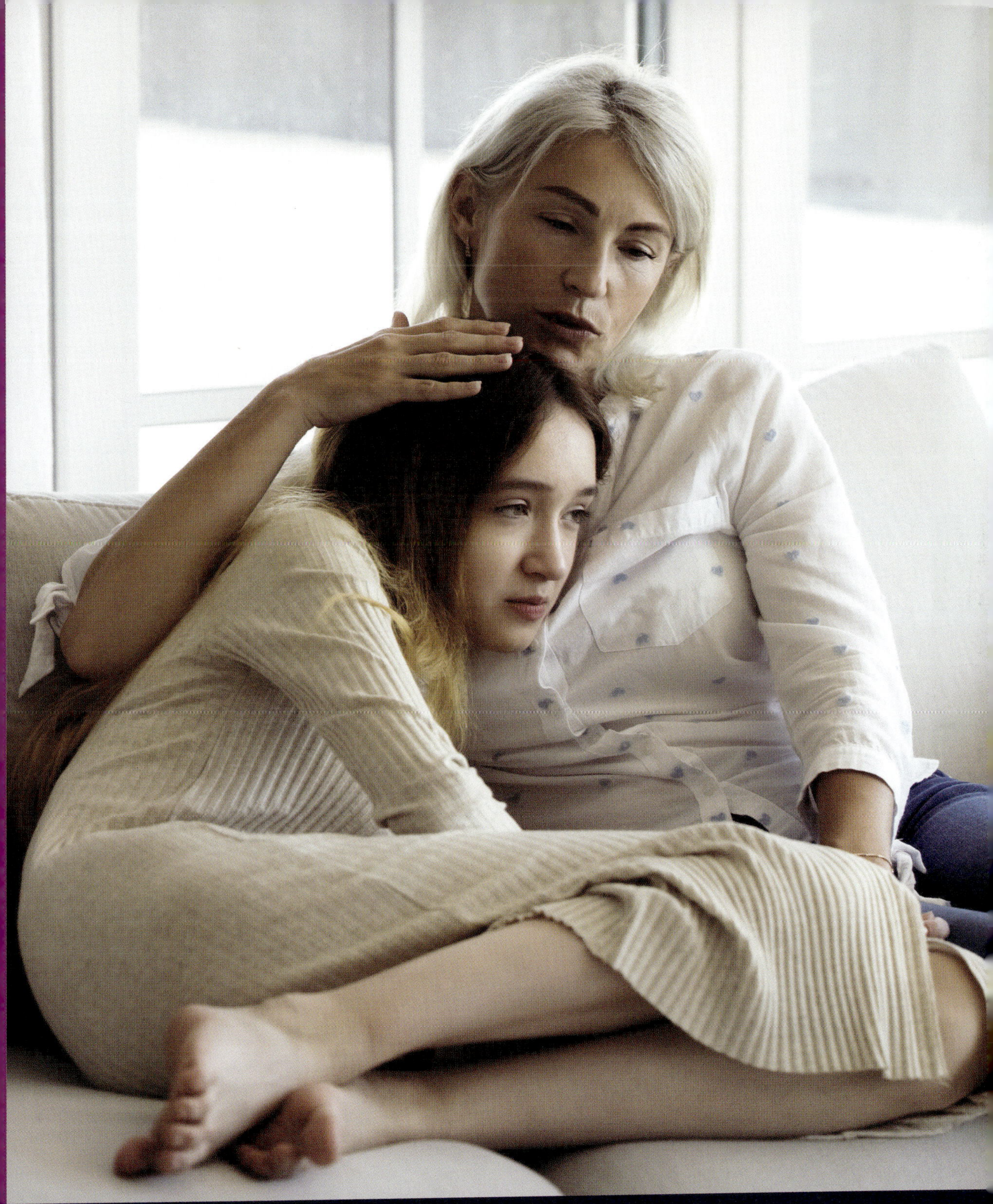

A REAL PROBLEM

Social anxiety disorder is a mental health condition, or mental illness. People might try to tell someone with a mental illness that their problems are all in their head. However, just because mental illnesses deal with the mind, that doesn't mean the problems they cause aren't real.

Mental health is just as important as physical health. Mental illnesses are just as **serious** as physical illnesses, such as cancer or the flu. They affect nearly 1 billion people around the world, and many don't have the support they need to get better.

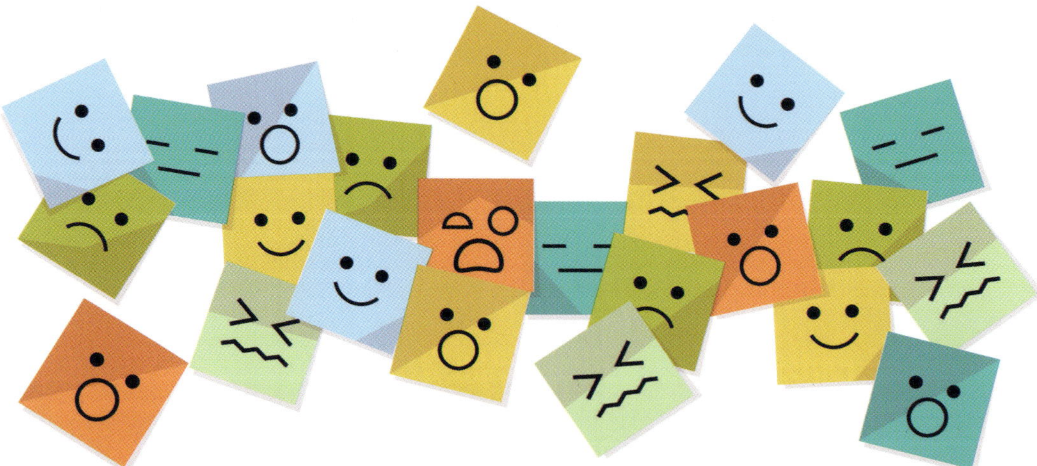

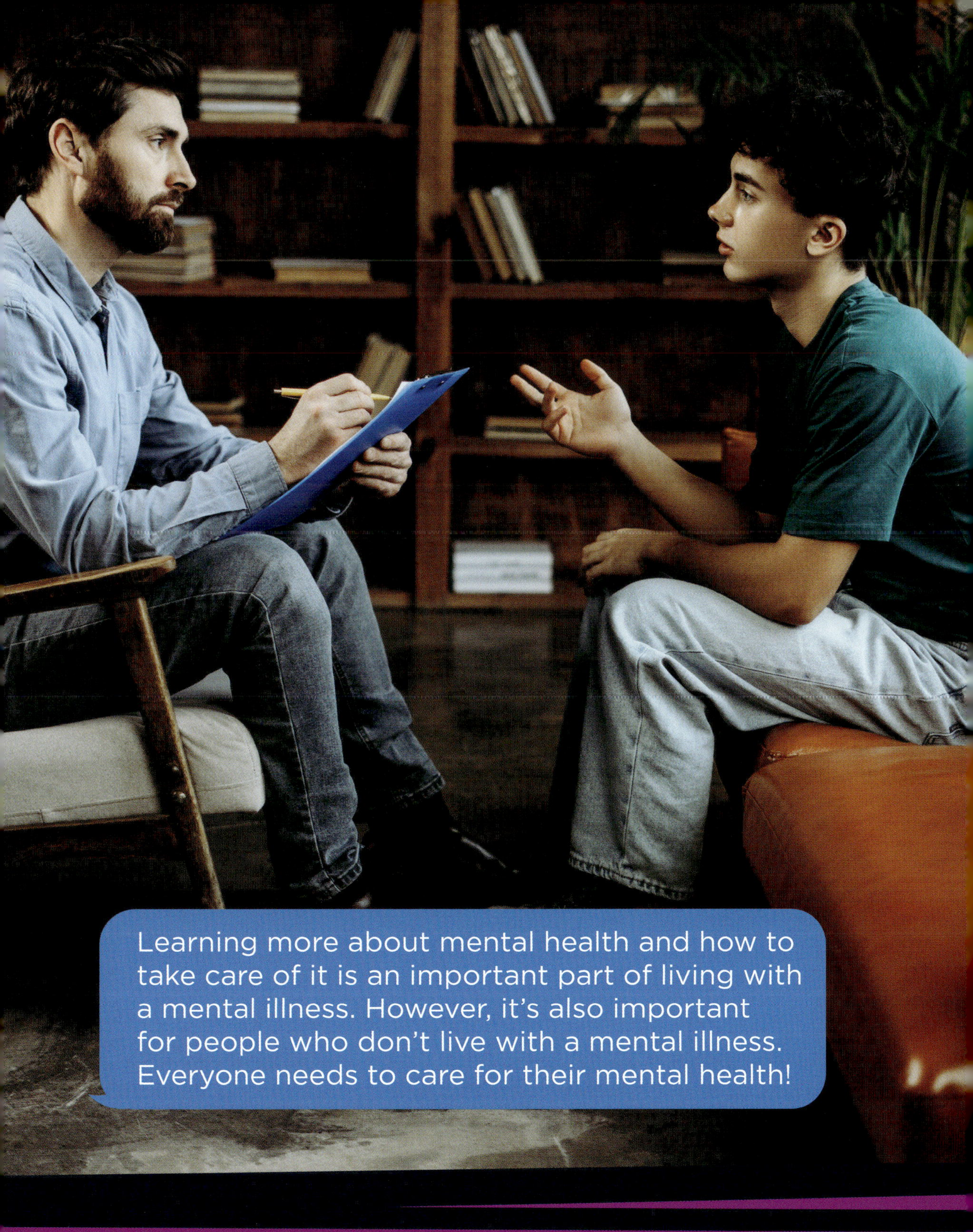

Learning more about mental health and how to take care of it is an important part of living with a mental illness. However, it's also important for people who don't live with a mental illness. Everyone needs to care for their mental health!

WHAT ARE ANXIETY DISORDERS?

Social anxiety disorder is part of a group of mental health conditions known as anxiety disorders. These are disorders that cause a person to feel more fear or worry than is considered normal for a certain situation. This fear or worry makes it hard for a person to do everyday tasks.

There are many kinds of anxiety disorders. Social anxiety disorder is one. Another is generalized anxiety disorder (GAD). Someone with GAD is constantly worried or afraid about things in their daily life, such as their grades or their family.

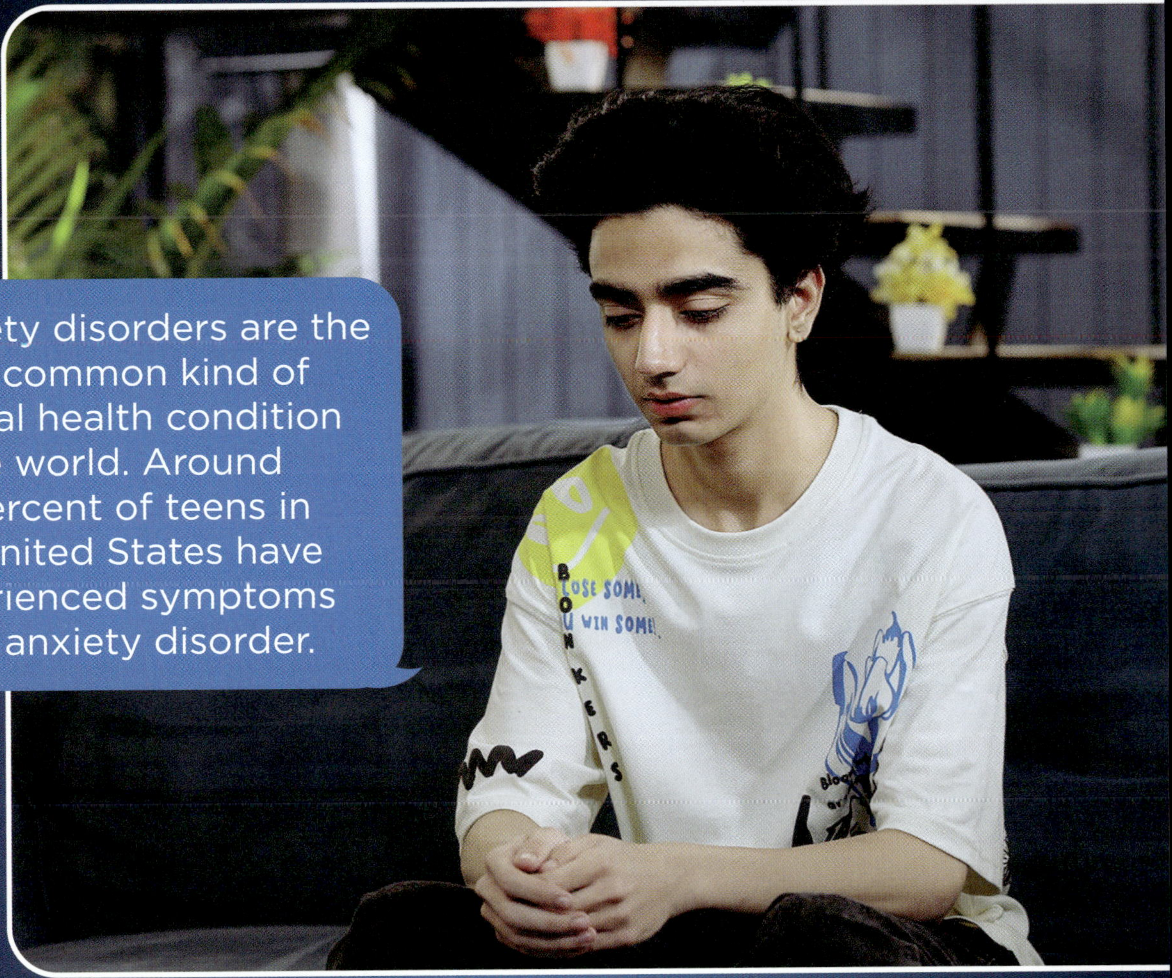

Anxiety disorders are the most common kind of mental health condition in the world. Around 20 percent of teens in the United States have experienced symptoms of an anxiety disorder.

WHAT CAUSES ANXIETY?

Scientists don't know exactly what causes anxiety disorders. However, they do believe certain neurotransmitters, which are chemicals that send messages between nerve cells, play a part. They also believe that certain parts of the brain are more active in people who have an anxiety disorder. In addition, many scientists think anxiety disorders have a genetic component, which means they could be passed from parent to child.

SOCIAL PHOBIA

Another kind of anxiety disorder is a specific phobia. This is an overpowering fear of a certain thing or situation. Social anxiety disorder is also known as social phobia because it deals with an extreme fear of social situations.

Everyone has things that make them feel afraid. However, a phobia is more than a normal fear. Someone with a phobia often does whatever they can to avoid the cause of their fear. If they can't avoid it, they **experience** extreme anxiety.

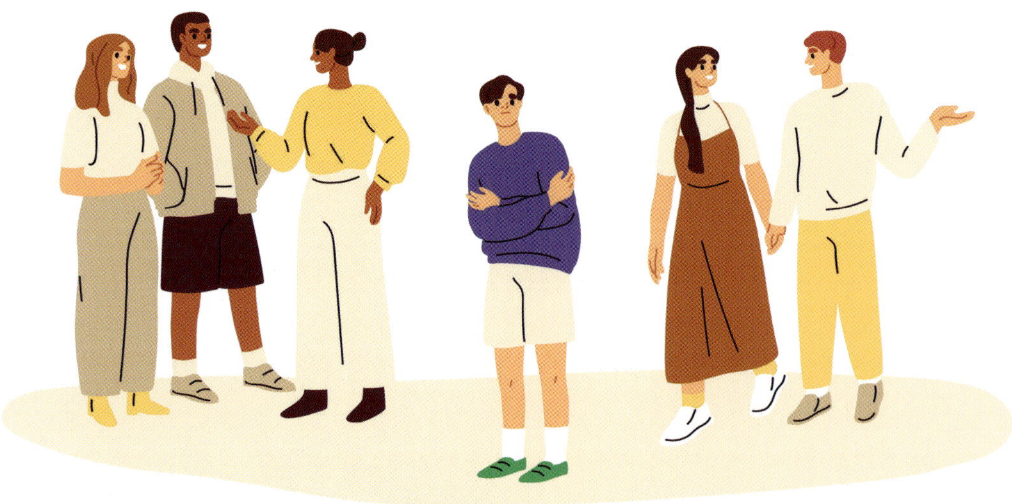

Fast Fact!

A specific phobia often shows up in childhood, often before the age of 10. However, people of all ages have specific phobias.

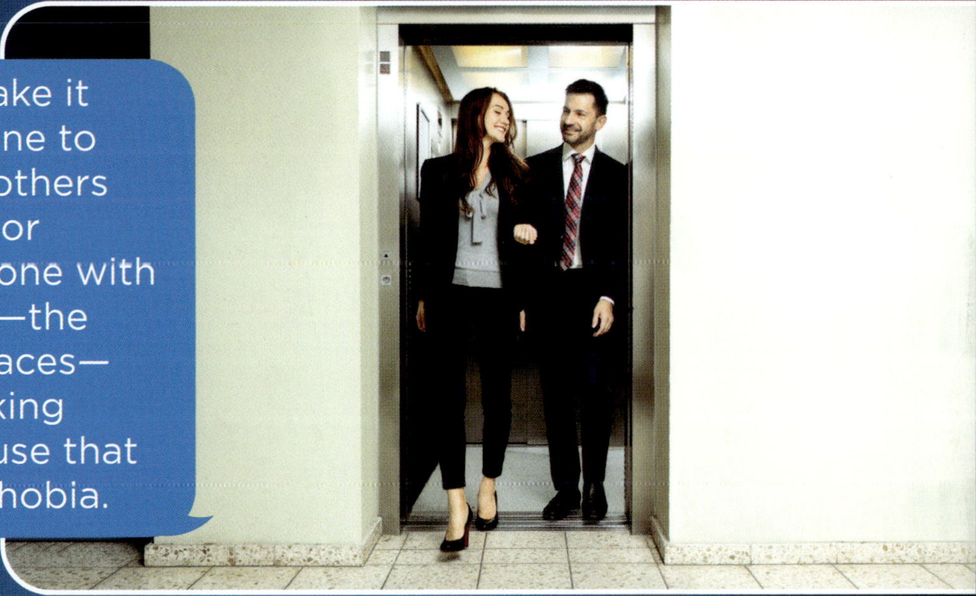

Phobias can make it hard for someone to do things that others can do easily. For example, someone with claustrophobia—the fear of tight spaces—might avoid taking elevators because that triggers their phobia.

COMMON SPECIFIC PHOBIAS

- fear of spiders
- fear of snakes
- fear of heights
- fear of thunderstorms
- fear of water
- fear of flying in an airplane
- fear of the dark
- fear of needles
- fear of blood
- fear of clowns

DON'T IGNORE IT!

Some people don't take their mental health seriously. They ignore the symptoms and don't get the **treatment** they need. This can cause lifelong problems—just like ignoring a physical health problem can.

For example, social anxiety disorder can cause loneliness if it's not treated. This can lead to **depression** or a substance use disorder. Someone with a substance use disorder uses or abuses a substance, such as alcohol or another drug, in a way that is known to be harmful.

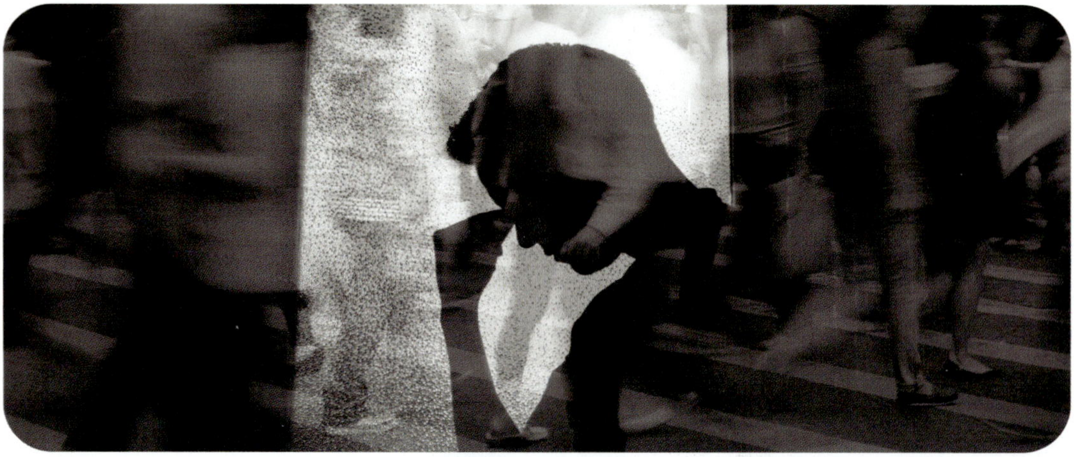

Fast Fact!

Many studies have shown that women are more likely than men to report living with social anxiety disorder.

When someone is living with two mental health disorders—such as depression and social anxiety—at the same time, it's called a comorbidity.

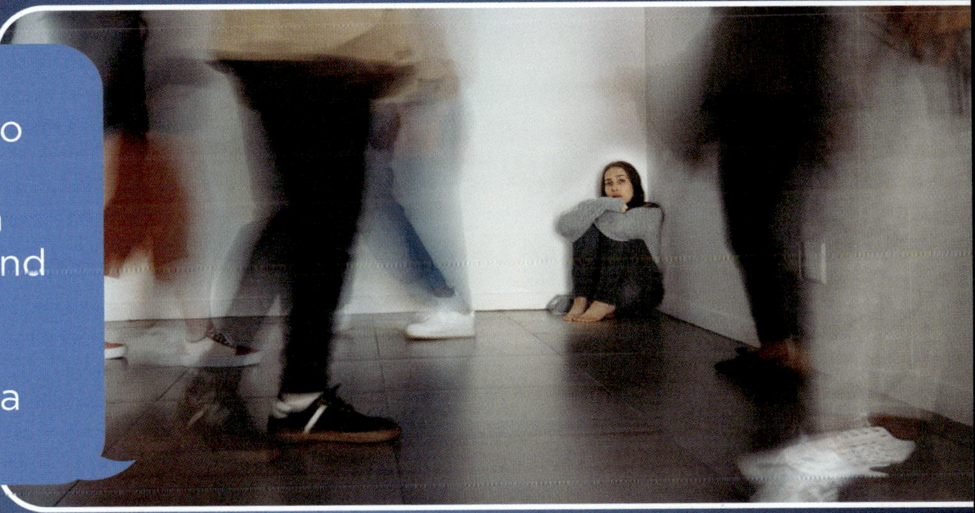

FOR MORE INFORMATION

Visit the following websites to learn more about mental health and mental illnesses:

National Alliance on Mental Illness: *www.nami.org*

Substance Abuse and Mental Health Services Administration: *www.samhsa.gov*

TeensHealth: *kidshealth.org/en/teens/your-mind*

The Trevor Project: *www.thetrevorproject.org/resources/category/mental-health*

Chapter 3

TREATING SOCIAL ANXIETY

When someone is living with social anxiety disorder, it may seem like things will never get better. However, there are treatments that can help people with social anxiety disorder.

The first step toward feeling better is asking for help. That often leads to getting a diagnosis. This is a formal statement from a doctor that someone has a medical condition. After someone is diagnosed with social anxiety disorder, they can start talking with their doctor about what treatment might work best for them.

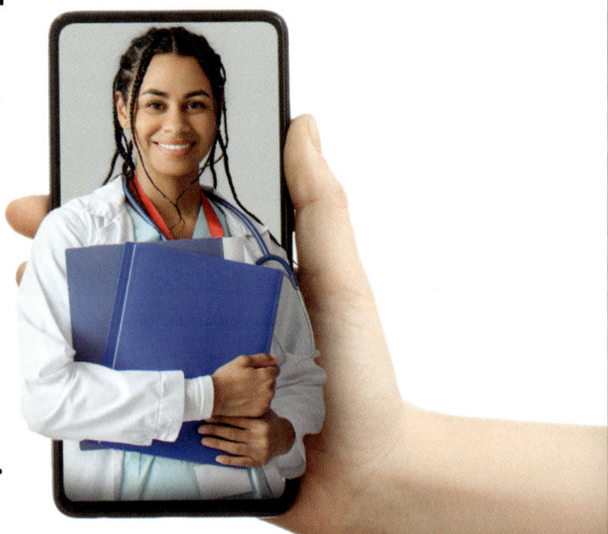

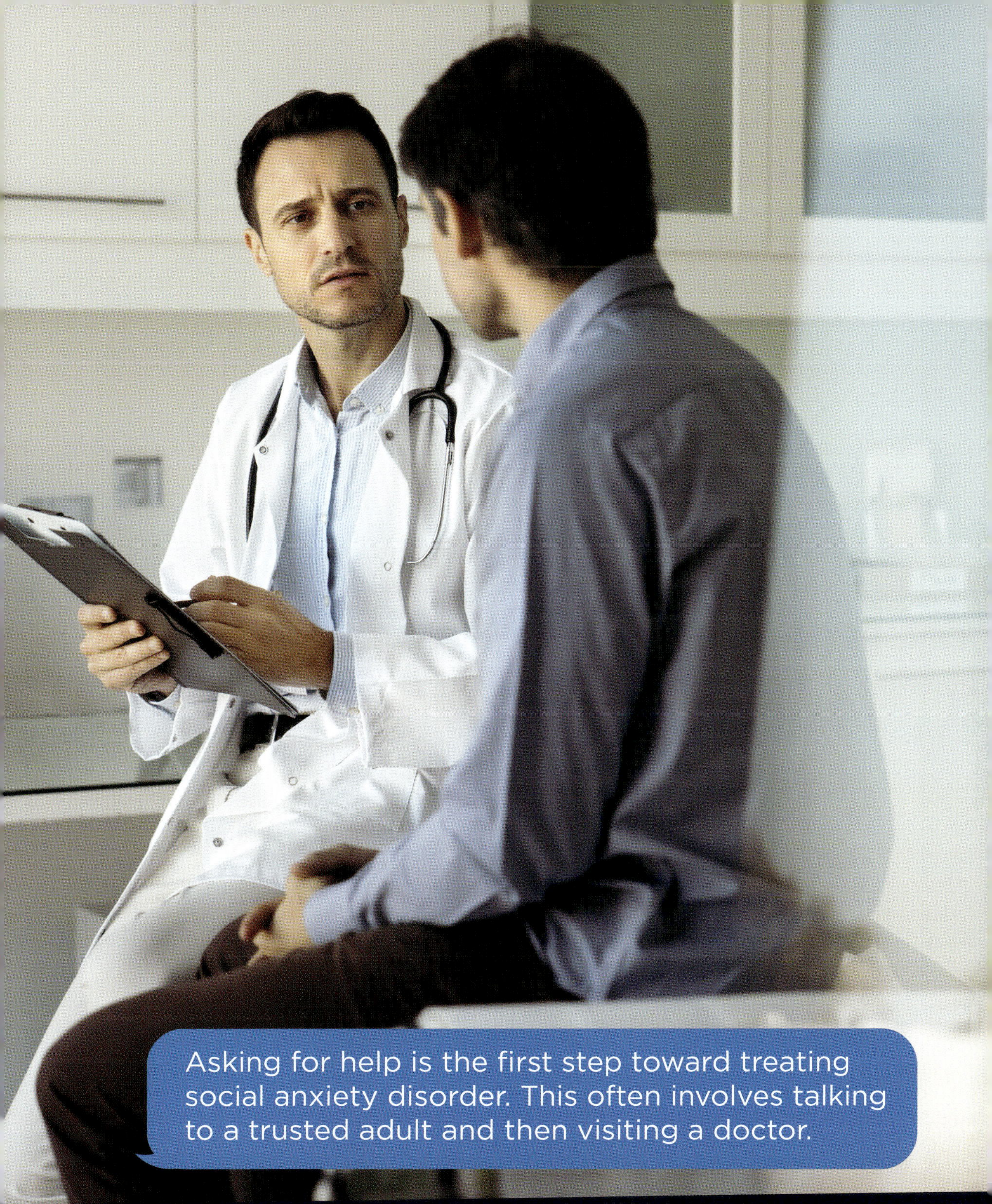

Asking for help is the first step toward treating social anxiety disorder. This often involves talking to a trusted adult and then visiting a doctor.

SEEING A THERAPIST

One of the most successful forms of treatment for social anxiety disorder is psychotherapy, or talk therapy. This kind of treatment involves talking to a therapist, who is trained to help people with their mental health.

Cognitive behavioral therapy (CBT) is the most common kind of therapy used to treat social anxiety disorder. CBT deals with changing negative thoughts and behaviors, which are ways of acting. CBT can help people with social anxiety disorder feel more **confident** in social situations.

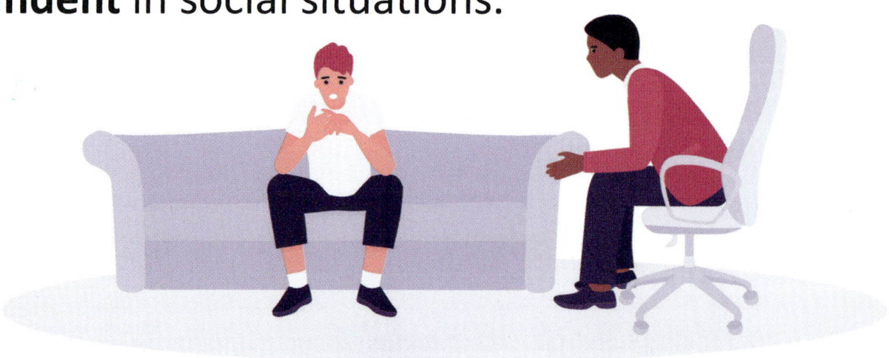

Fast Fact!

In some cases, exposure therapy is used for people with social anxiety disorder. This kind of therapy allows people to face their fears in a controlled, safe way and learn to handle them with confidence. For example, someone with social anxiety disorder might practice talking on the phone to cope with their fears.

CBT is most often done for a set number of weeks. After that, the **patient** has learned enough to manage their mental health on their own. However, some people need—or want—to continue to see a therapist for months or even years.

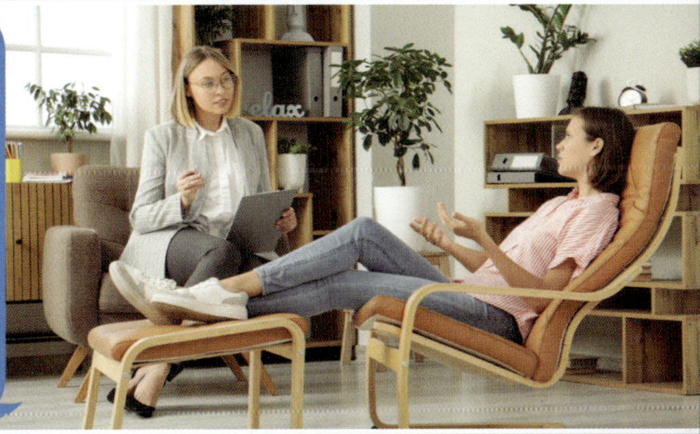

FOR MORE INFORMATION

Here are some helpful workbooks that you can use to practice CBT skills at home:

David, Lee, and Debbie Brewin. *10 Minutes to Beat Anxiety and Panic.* London, UK: Jessica Kingsley Publishers, 2025.

Shannon, Jennifer. *The Shyness and Social Anxiety Workbook for Teens.* Oakland, CA: Instant Help Books, 2022.

Walker, Bridget Flynn. *Social Anxiety Relief for Teens.* Oakland, CA: New Harbinger Publications, 2021.

MENTAL HEALTH MEDICATIONS

Some people have success treating their social anxiety disorder with CBT alone. Others, however, need extra help. This often comes in the form of medication, or drugs, used to treat mental illnesses.

The most common group of drugs used to treat social anxiety disorder are selective serotonin reuptake inhibitors (SSRIs). They work by increasing the amount of serotonin in the brain. Serotonin is a neurotransmitter that plays a big part in a person's mood. SSRIs used to treat social anxiety disorder include Zoloft, Prozac, and Lexapro.

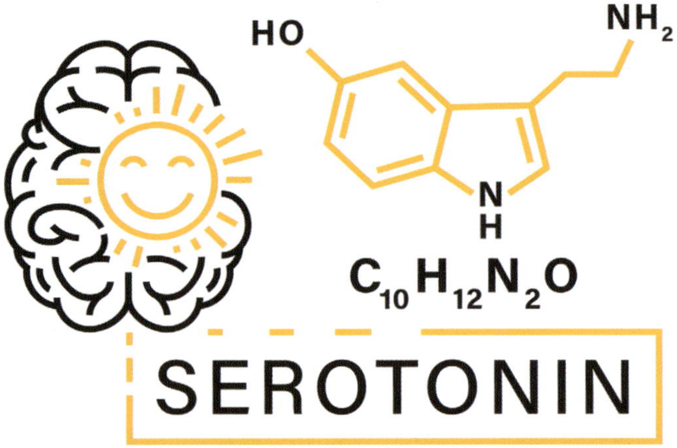

Not all medications used to treat social anxiety disorder are safe for teenagers to use. It's important to only take medication that your doctor has said is safe.

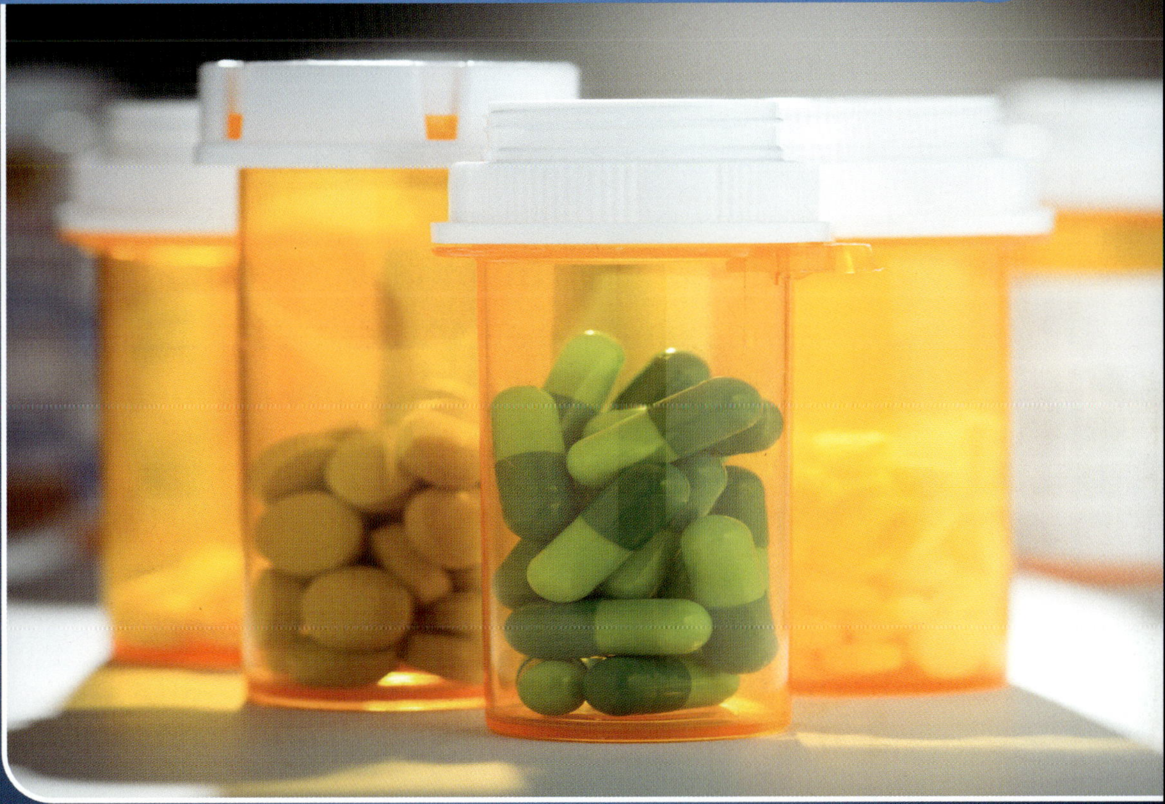

OTHER OPTIONS

Some other medications can also be used to treat social anxiety disorder. They include medications called SNRIs that increase the amount of serotonin and norepinephrine in a person's brain. Norepinephrine is another neurotransmitter. It plays a part in how we deal with **stress**. Beta blockers are another group of drugs used to treat social anxiety. They help stop physical symptoms of anxiety, such as shaking hands or a fast heartbeat.

TRIAL AND ERROR

Taking medicine for a mental illness is no different than taking medicine for any other health problem. However, finding the right mental health medication isn't always easy.

One drug might not work or might have side effects that are too hard to live with. Then, the patient has to try a different one. This can happen over and over until the right medication and dosage, or amount, is found. It can be hard work, but feeling better is worth it.

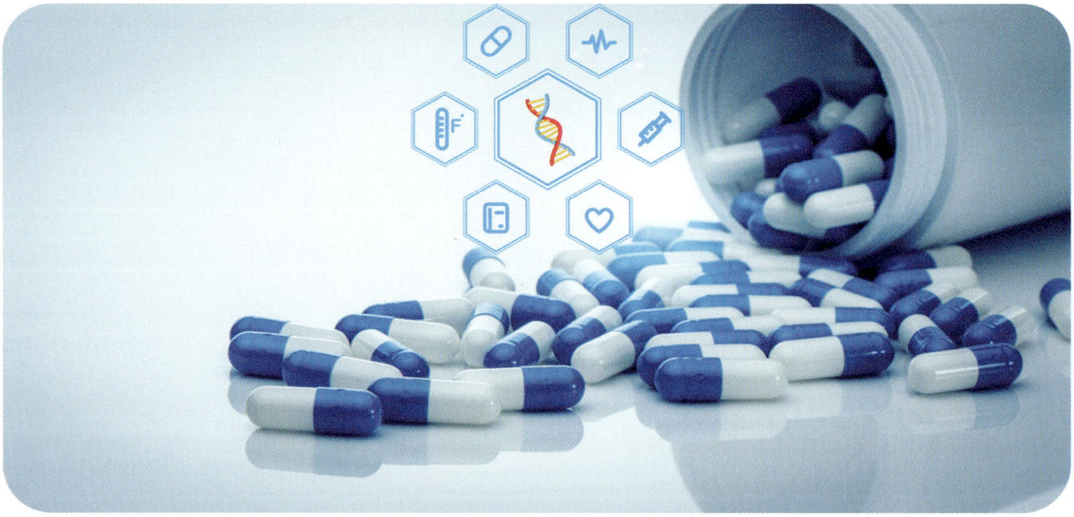

Fast Fact!

Psychiatrists and psychologists are both doctors that treat people's mental health. The main difference between them is that psychiatrists are medical doctors and psychologists aren't. This means psychologists can't give people medication to treat their mental health.

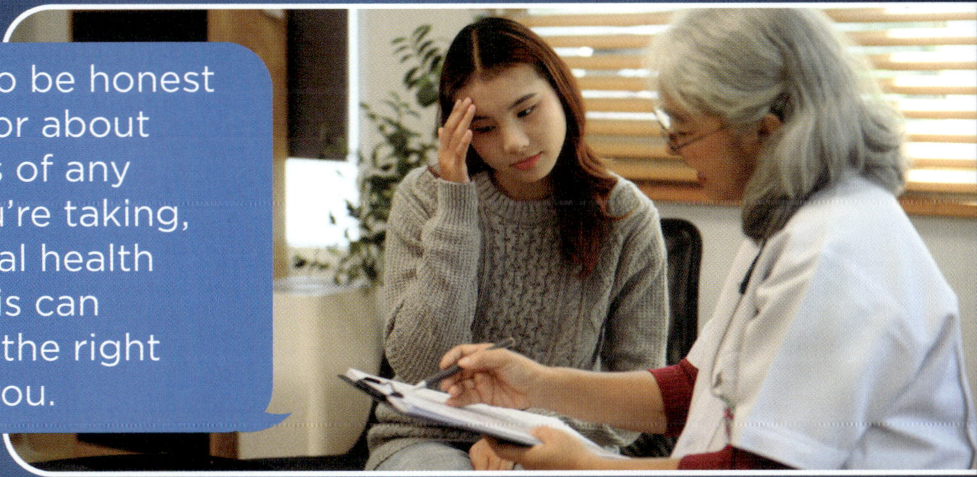

It's important to be honest with your doctor about the side effects of any medication you're taking, including mental health medication. This can help them find the right treatment for you.

SIDE EFFECTS

Common side effects of SSRIs and other mental health medications include:

- stomach problems
- problems with sleep
- headaches
- dry mouth
- increased anxiety
- sleepiness
- changes in weight

Feeling Like Myself

I've struggled with anxiety ever since I was in middle school. It was getting really bad, so I started seeing a therapist. Therapy gave me new **coping** skills, but I was still feeling anxious most of the time. My psychiatrist said I could also try taking medication to treat my anxiety.

At first, I was scared. What if it made me feel worse? What if I didn't feel like myself anymore? But I knew I couldn't keep feeling so anxious.

The first drug I tried made me really tired, so Dr. Lee had me try a different one. I've been taking that one for almost a year now, and I feel so much better. I finally feel like myself again!

Many people continue seeing a therapist after starting to take medication for their mental health. Doctors believe those two kinds of treatments often work best when used together.

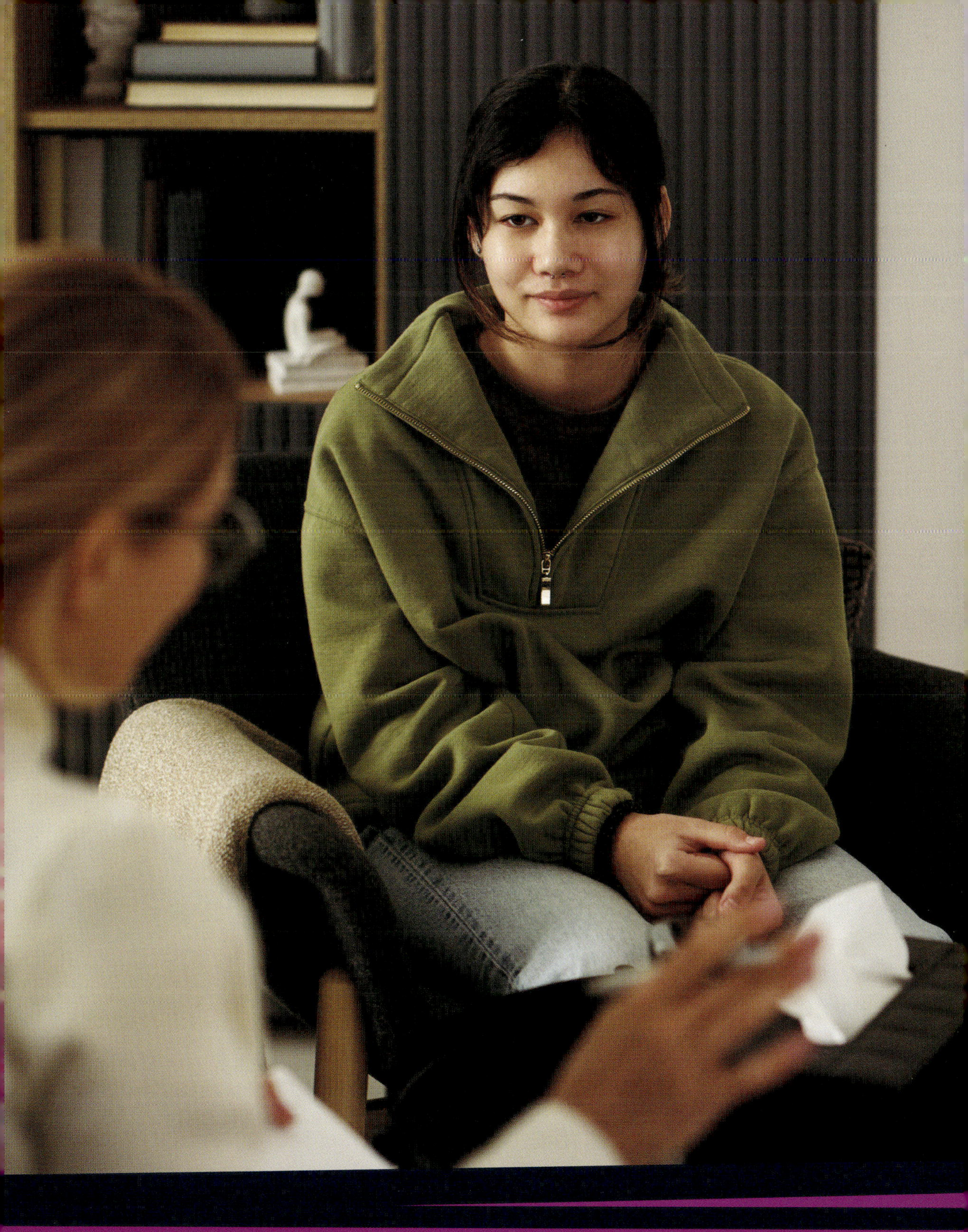

Chapter 4

LIVING WITH SOCIAL ANXIETY

Medication and therapy are important ways to treat social anxiety disorder. However, there are also other things people can do to help their mental health.

For example, moving your body can help your mental health. Finding a kind of movement that makes you feel good—whether it's playing a sport, dancing around the house, or lifting weights—can improve both your physical and mental health. In addition, it's important to drink enough water and eat enough. Eating a variety of foods is also helpful for overall health.

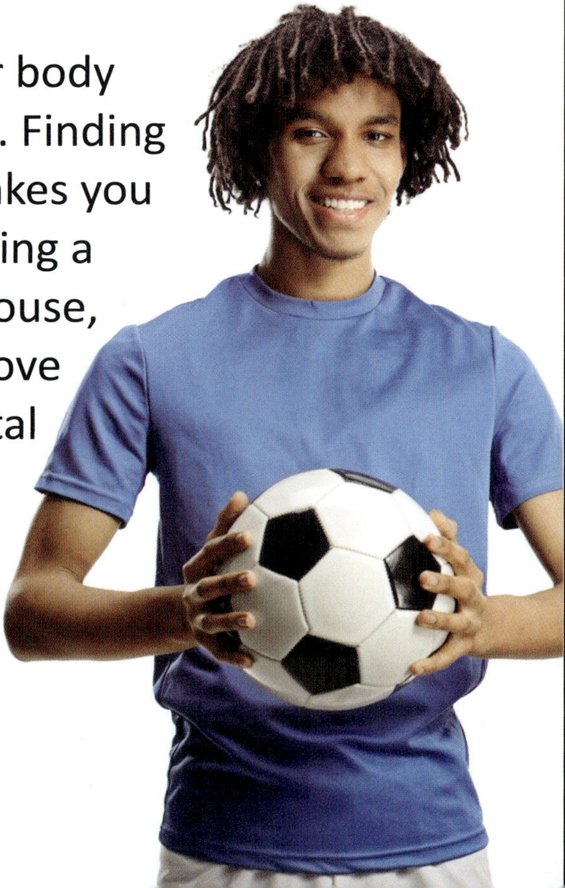

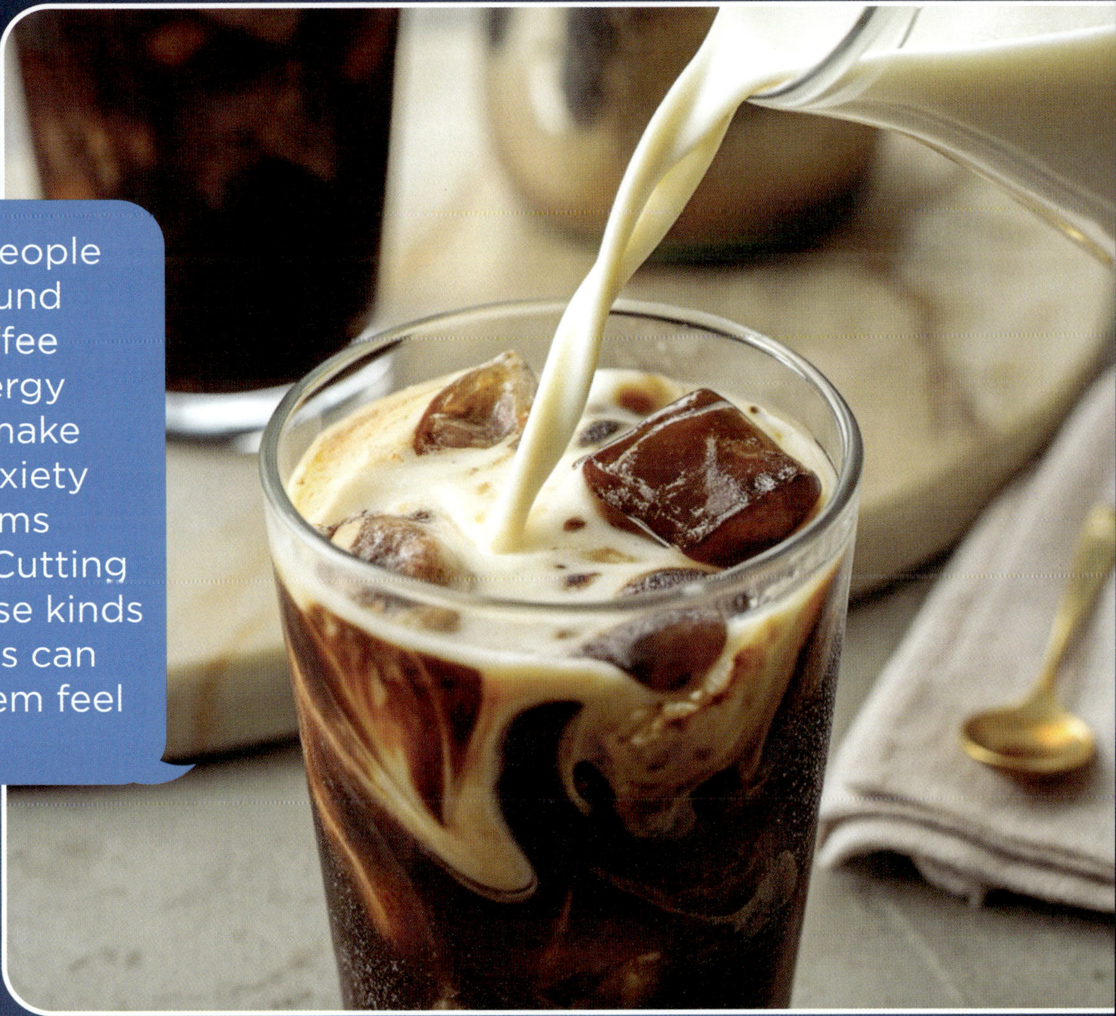

Some people have found that coffee and energy drinks make their anxiety symptoms worse. Cutting out those kinds of drinks can help them feel better.

WHO TO TRUST?

It's common to see videos on social media of influencers talking about things they eat, drink, or buy to help them feel their best. They might say a certain diet is helping "cure" their anxiety or that a **supplement** treated their depression. However, it's important to remember that you shouldn't take medical advice from strangers on the internet. Talk to your doctor instead.

TAKE A BREATH

Taking slow, deep breaths can help you stay calm in stressful situations. **Focusing** on your breathing can also ground you in what's really happening in the moment. That can help you stop worrying about what will happen. This is called being mindful.

Mindful movement and breathing are at the heart of yoga. People who practice yoga hold their body in certain poses while focusing on their breathing. Yoga can be very helpful for people with anxiety.

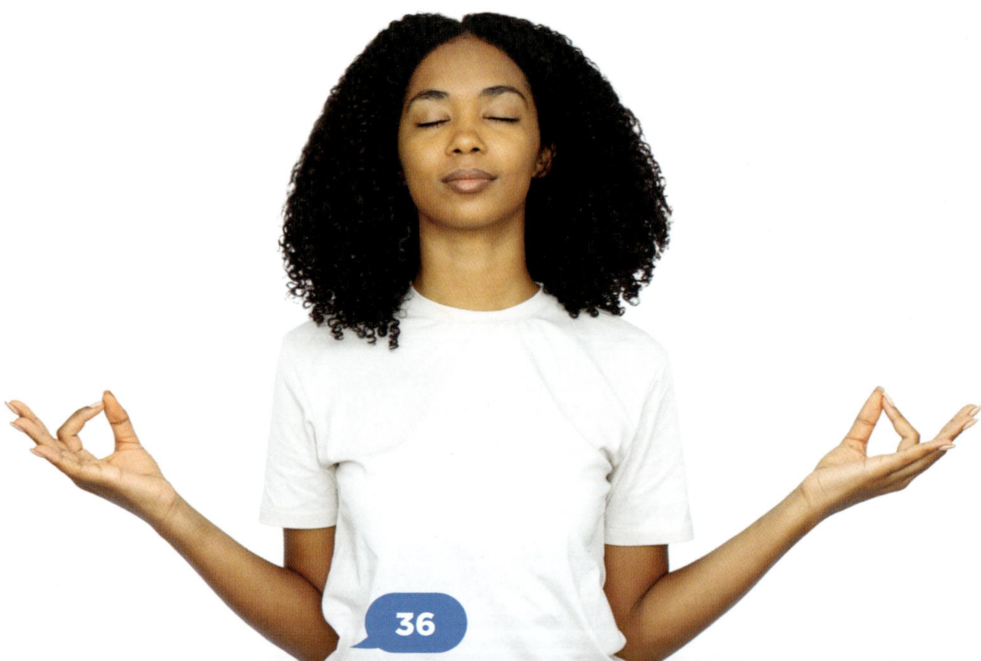

Yoga and meditation have become popular practices in the 21st century. However, people have been practicing them since ancient times!

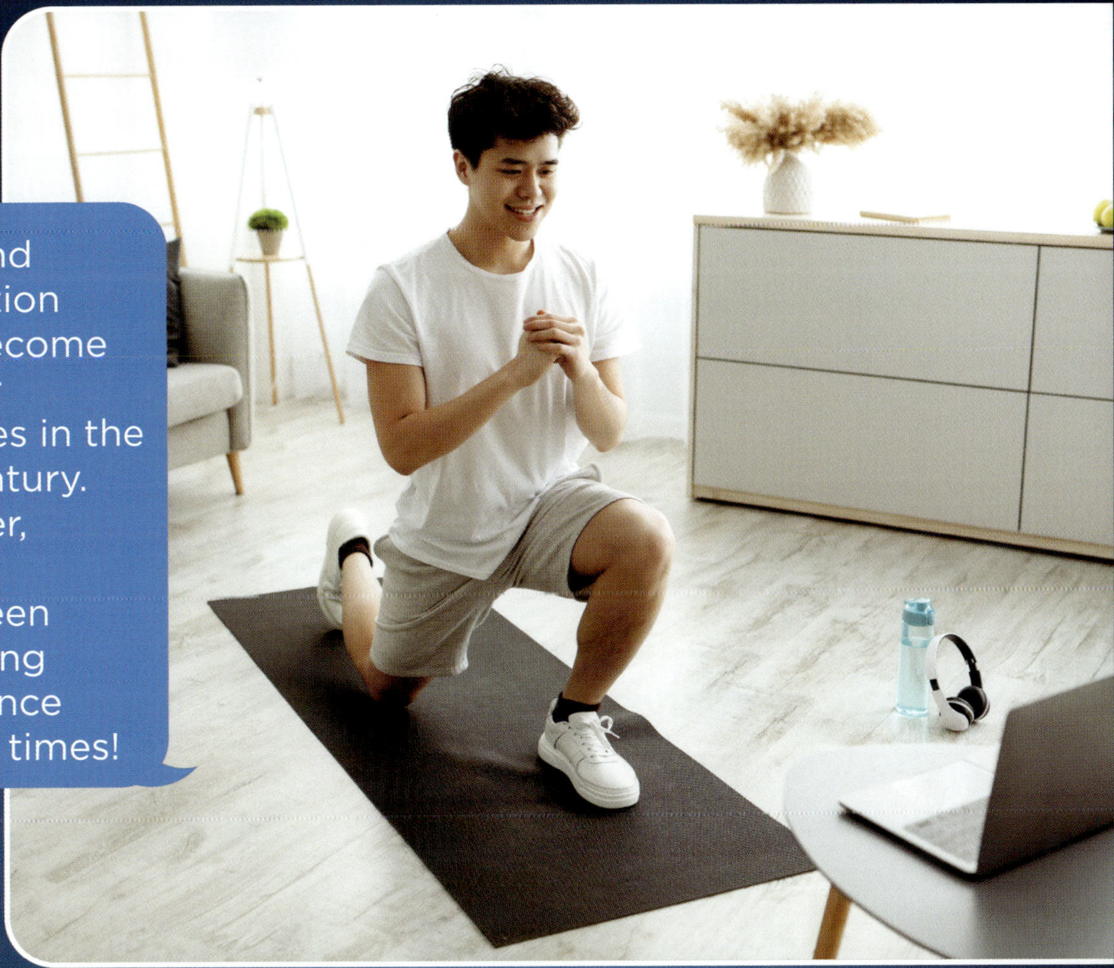

LET'S MEDITATE!

Many people who have anxiety practice meditation to help them feel better. When someone meditates, they try to focus on their breathing, a peaceful saying or sound, or how their body feels. This allows them to let go of racing or stressful thoughts. In some cases, meditation also involves focusing on feelings of loving kindness toward yourself and others. Meditation can be a helpful tool for coping with anxiety and building confidence.

PATIENCE AND PRACTICE

Coping with social anxiety disorder isn't easy. It takes a lot of bravery to ask for help and a lot of strength to do the work needed to treat the disorder. It also takes patience, because change doesn't happen overnight. Finding the right medication, doing the work in therapy, and practicing new coping skills in social situations take time.

An important part of dealing with any mental illness is showing self-compassion. This means treating yourself kindly, even when things are hard.

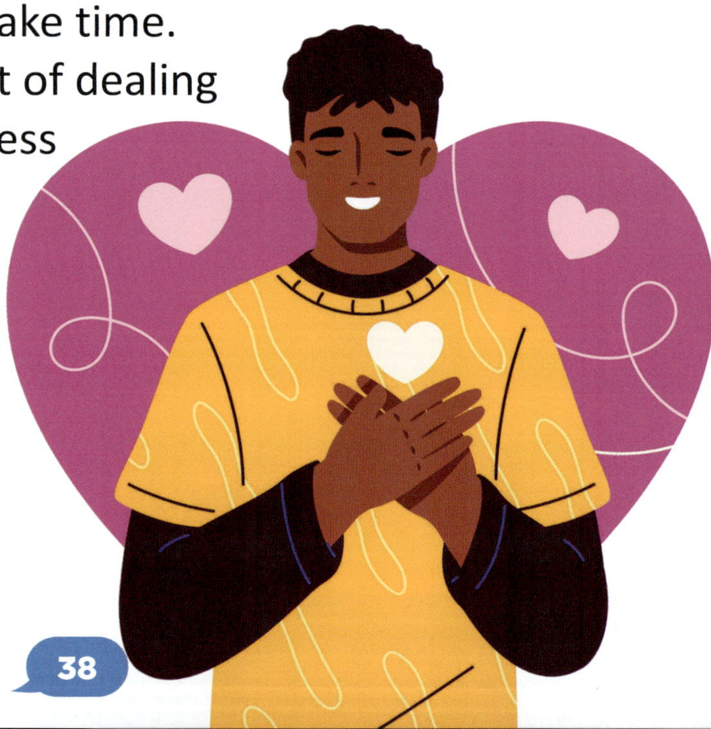

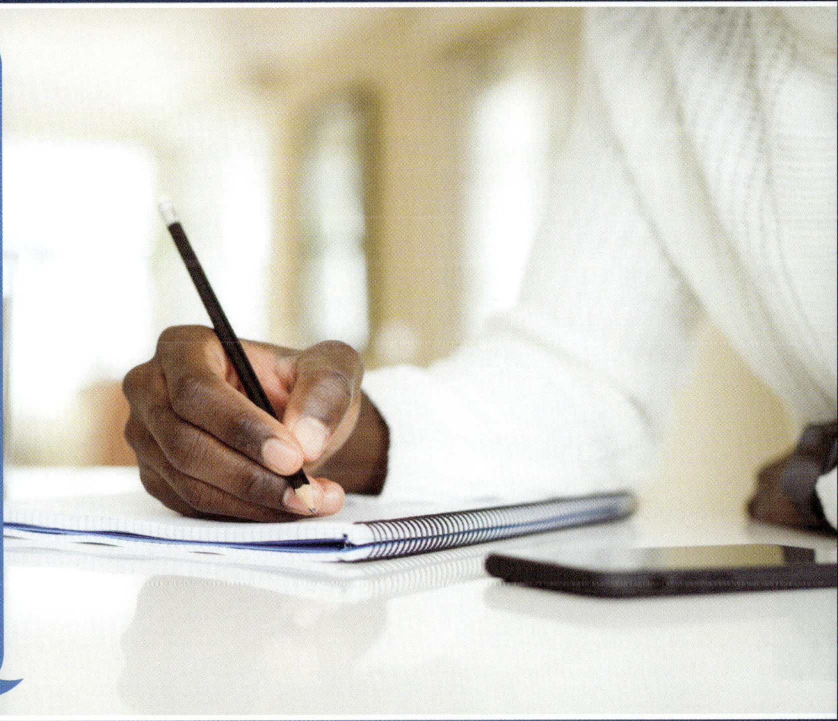

Practicing self-compassion means not beating yourself up if you have a bad day. It's going to happen! That's why it's important to celebrate good days. One way to do this is by writing about them in a journal. Journaling is good for mental health.

WAYS TO PRACTICE

Here are some ways to practice coping with social anxiety. These are good to try as you make progress with therapy or medication (or both). It can be helpful to have a trusted friend or family member around for support when you do these for the first time.

- Ask for help finding something at a store.
- Go out to eat with a trusted friend or family member, and eat in front of them.
- Say hello to someone.
- Give someone a compliment.
- Call a trusted friend or family member on the phone.

HOW TO HELP

People often want to help a loved one living with social anxiety, but they don't always know how. The best way to start is by learning more. This can involve reading about social anxiety disorder. It can also be as simple as actively listening when someone with social anxiety disorder is telling you how they feel.

Being patient with someone with social anxiety is also important. Don't judge them for having a hard time or tell them to stop worrying. This might make them feel worse.

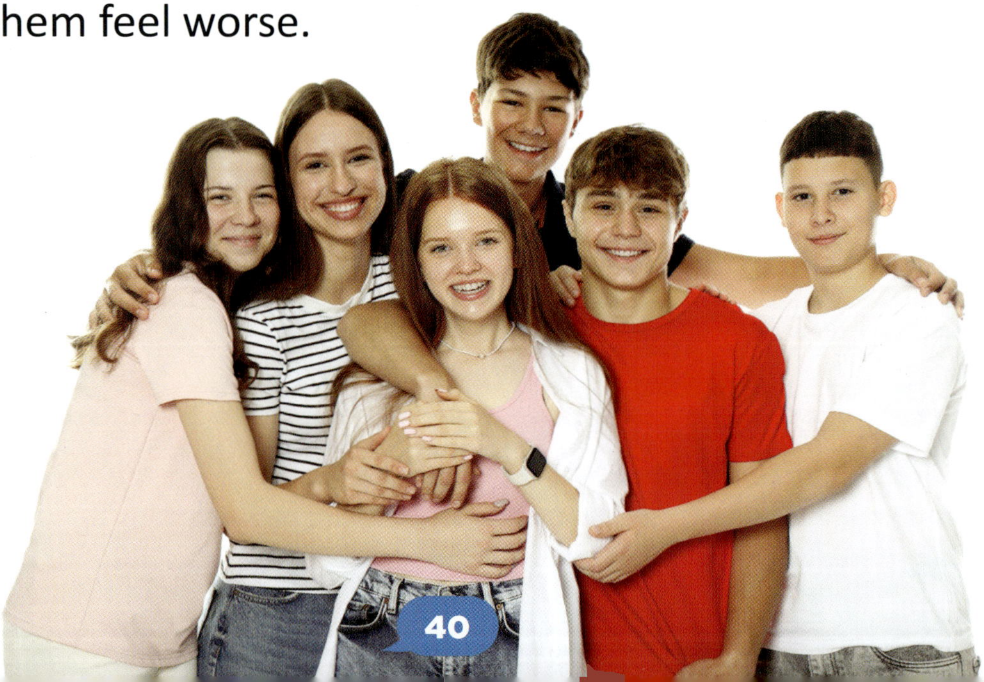

Fast Fact!

LGBTQIA+ young people are more likely than their peers to experience mental health problems such as social anxiety disorder.

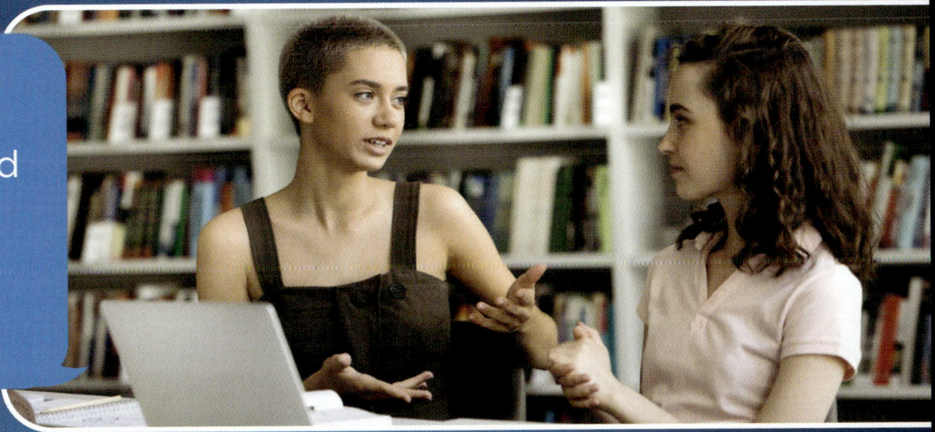

People with social anxiety disorder are generally afraid of being judged by others. Being a supportive friend can be a big help.

FOR MORE INFORMATION

The following books can help you learn more about social anxiety disorder:

Harts, Shannon H. *Stress and Anxiety.* Buffalo, NY: Rosen Publishing, 2021.

Lorenz, Sarah Jo. *Anxiety Disorders.* Hollywood, FL: Mason Crest, 2023.

McManus, Celina. *Understanding Anxiety.* San Diego: CA: BrightPoint Press, 2021.

Miller, Verity. *I Get Panic Attacks ... What's Next?* Buffalo, NY: Rosen Publishing, 2022.

REASONS TO HOPE

Living with social anxiety disorder can make people feel hopeless. However, there are plenty of reasons to hope. With the help of therapy, medication, or some mix of both, most people with social anxiety disorder are able to manage their anxiety. This allows them to enjoy social situations instead of fearing them.

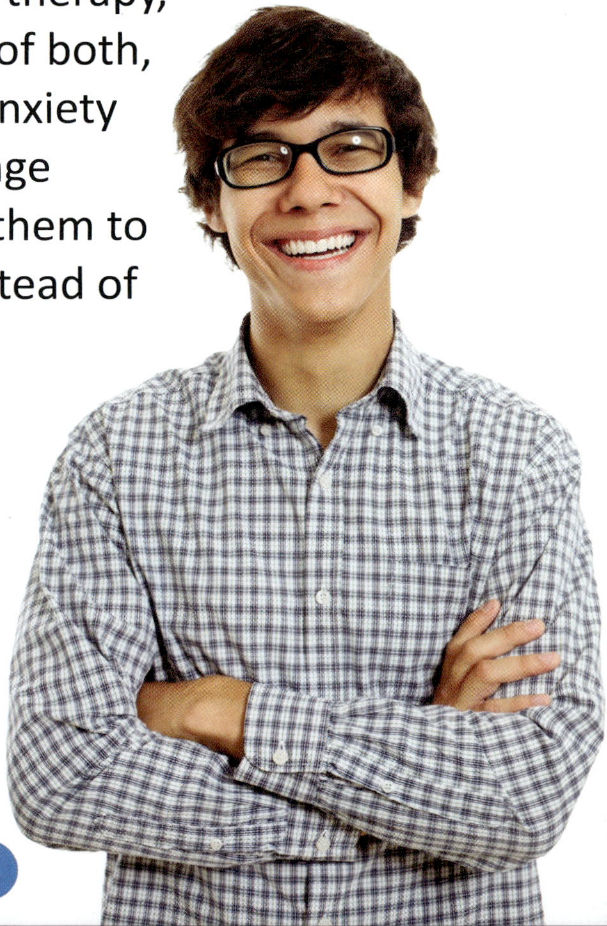

If you think you might be dealing with social anxiety, reach out to someone you trust. Asking for help might seem scary, but it's the best thing you can do for your mental health.

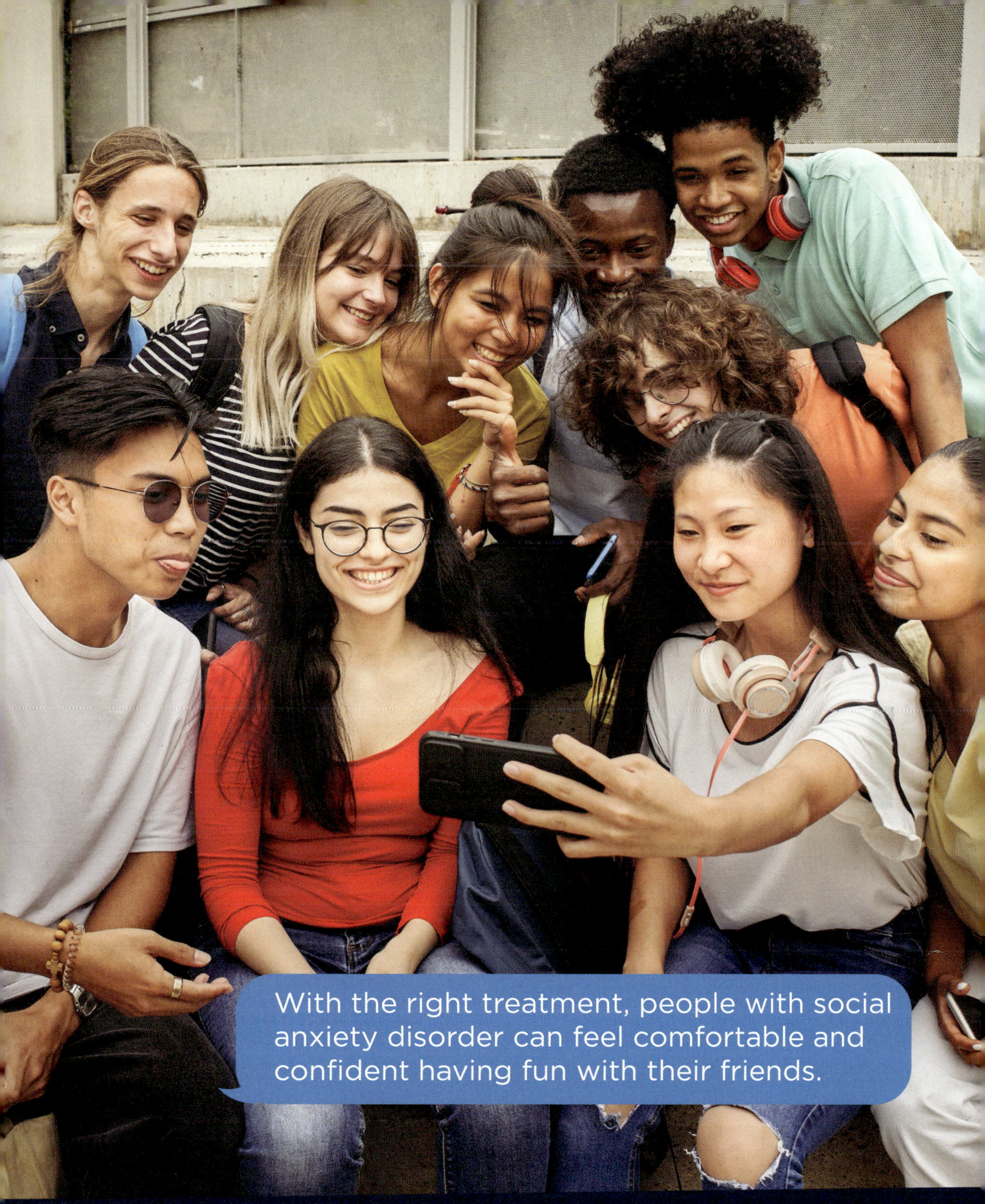

With the right treatment, people with social anxiety disorder can feel comfortable and confident having fun with their friends.

Having Fun Again

I was scared to tell my mom about how anxious I'd been feeling. But I knew she would help me.

My mom took me to the doctor, and Dr. Grant said I have social anxiety disorder. It feels good to have a name for what I've been feeling.

I started seeing a therapist, and it's been really good for me. I do my therapy homework, and it's helping me feel a lot better. Sometimes I still get nervous about going to school, especially on days when I know I have to talk in front of the class. But I don't feel sick anymore. I know my friends are there to support me, and I'm excited to hang out with them!

Everyone feels anxious sometimes, but it doesn't have to take over your life!

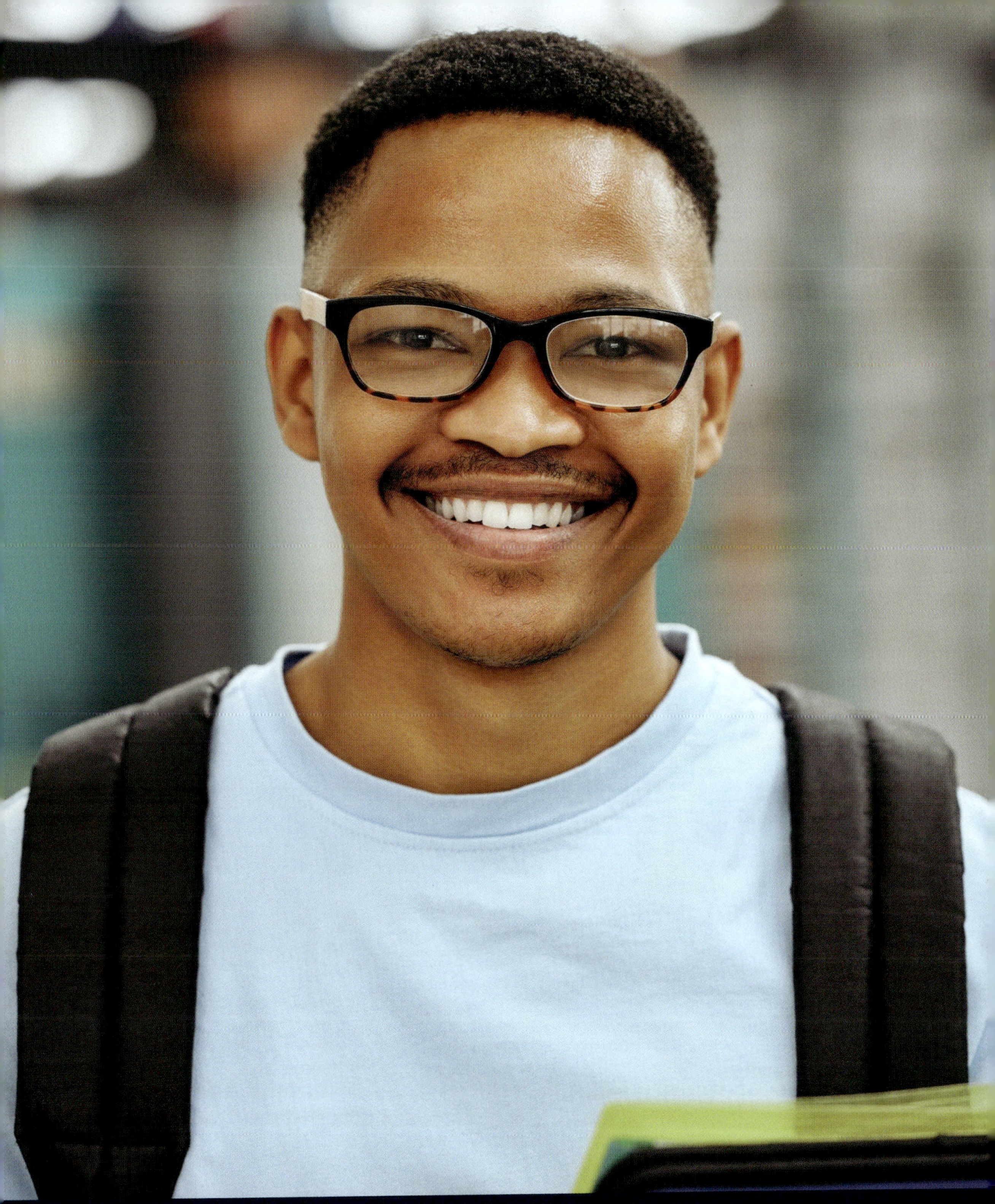

GLOSSARY

awkward: Clumsy or not confident, especially around other people.

confident: Having a feeling of belief that you can do something well.

cope: To try to manage with some success.

depression: A mental health condition in which a person feels very sad, hopeless, and unimportant and is often unable to do basic tasks because of this.

embarrass: To cause a feeling of foolishness.

experience: To do or see something or to have something happen to you.

extreme: More than what is expected.

focus: To direct attention or effort at something.

interview: A formal meeting to gain information in order to decide if someone is qualified for a job.

irrational: Not based on reason.

mental: Dealing with the mind.

nausea: The feeling of having an upset stomach that often involves the urge to throw up.

normal: Usual.

patient: A person who receives care from a doctor.
physical: Dealing with the body.
serious: Causing worry or harm.
situation: All the facts, conditions, and events that affect someone or something in a certain time and place.
stress: A state of strong feelings of worry.
supplement: Something taken in by the body to supply more of something that is needed.
treatment: Care given to a person that is sick or hurt.
trigger: To make something start to happen.

INDEX